W9-DAX-218

SPACE HEART

SPACE HEART

A MEMOIR IN STAGES

LINDA BUCKMASTER

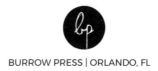

BURROW PRESS | ORLANDO, FL

© Linda Buckmaster, 2018.
All rights reserved.

Published by Burrow Press
PO Box 533709
Orlando, FL 32853
burrowpress.com

ISBN: 978-1-941681-73-2
LCCN: 2018943468

Book Design: Ryan Rivas

Cover Art © Joan Proudman, 2018.
joanproudman.com

This publication is made possible in part by our Founding Sponsors:

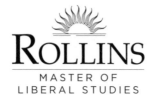

Burrow Press thrives on the direct support of its subscribers, and generous support from grants, companies, foundations, and individuals.

 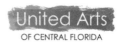

To the memory of
my mother, who always knew I would write a book;
my father, who should have written one;
and my little brother, who I never thought I would write about.

STAGE I: LAUNCHED

STAGE II: FALLOUT

STAGE III: RECOVERY

STAGE I: LAUNCHED

Now we have parallel [rocket] staging. The two boosters and the main engine are running simultaneously. Our total thrust can easily be combined adding up the three [stage] thrust sources:

$$kF_{*,tot} = m'_{p,i} \cdot v_{*,i}$$
$$\sum_{i=1}^{} F_{*,tot} = m'_{Vulcain} \cdot v_{*,Vulcain} + 2 \cdot m'_{P230} \cdot v_{*,P230} = 9{,}480{,}525N$$

-INSTITUTE OF ASTRONAUTICS, SPACECRAFT I

Let's light this firecracker.

-ALAN B. SHEPARD, WAITING FOR LAUNCH IN THE *FREEDOM* 7 CAPSULE

BARRIER ISLAND

The limestone shelf has always been here. Porous limestone, ancient fossil limestone, an African fragment broken from the great continent Pangea, forming a hard, swollen finger pointing south. Thin sea water, skinny as a snake, slips over the shelf, falling and rising for a hundred and forty million years. Glaciers creep close from the north; glaciers recede.

At the top of the finger, the wide Suwannee Channel cuts this new shelf off from the rest of the land mass. Eventually, time fills the channel with sediment and this fragment joins the continent. Quartz-rich Appalachian sand arrives from the north. Pushed by the water, the sand is always moving across the limestone. It scurries like pale crabs, filling in the low places, piling up against the high.

On the Atlantic side, along the middle of the coastline, a long, soft barrier island emerges like a slender, sleeping body. For miles, this island stretches lazily between swirling inlets on its north and south ends, where salt water rushes in with the tides and brackish lagoon water slides out. In the middle of the coastline, a cape of sand swells like a breast into the Atlantic— *Cabo Cañaveral,* as the Spanish call it, "place of canes." Tall cord grasses stand in the shallow salt marsh, sea oats send their stalks six feet high, and gray-green palmettos secure the wide dune of sand fronting the sea.

Here and there, coquina rock made of fragmented shells and quartz sits just offshore like rough armor. The sea pounds the east side of the beach in the winter and whispers in the summer. The shallow tidal lagoons languish, drifting south, as a river might. The rains pour down, but the land is so porous— limestone, sand, coquina—that the water disappears into it.

Sand and water waltz together under the relentless sun, unchanged for millennia, ignored, until the Rockets arrive.

SPACE HEART

I. On July 24, 1950, *Bumper V-2* blasts off a tiny, hand-poured cement pad in the middle of the palmettos to become the first rocket launched from Cape Canaveral. As my mother waits out the sticky final months of her pregnancy with me, two hundred miles down the coast in Miami, neither she nor my father realize this event will have anything to do with us, if they even hear about it. Although my father is studying electrical engineering on the GI Bill, he never imagines he will one day become a rocket engineer. In fact, no one can really foresee the new world that *Bumper* launches that humid morning.

Conditions are so primitive at the launch site that those working on it receive hazardous duty pay to compensate for the swamps, four species of poisonous snakes, and alligators. The aggressive saltmarsh mosquitoes that attack the scientists are able to reproduce up to a million offspring per square yard in one day. Bobcats and sleek Florida panthers roam the scrub. Cottonmouths, copperheads, and rattlers slither around estuaries, across coastal dunes, and through pine flatlands that sit just inches above the water table. Directions to the launch site posted along the sandy road include the admonition, "Don't stop or you'll bog down."

My mother's water breaks on the cusp of three hurricanes. September is prime hurricane season in Miami, and this year several circle her due date. Storms Charlie, Dog, and Easy bounce over the south Atlantic as my father carries my mother's suitcase onto the hospital elevator. When my mother wakes some time later, the hurricanes are veering away from Miami, and she has a new baby girl sleeping down the hall in the nursery.

She holds me in her lap as we ride in my father's 1946 Chevy along the narrow strip of asphalt that is Southwest Eighth Street, the Tamiami Trail, stretching a hundred and ten miles through the Everglades to Tampa on the west coast.

Our trailer park blooms lush and green with tropical vegetation. Raucous local birds and songbirds just arriving from up north fill the air. The heavy smells of night-blooming jasmine and gardenias hang in the humidity. My mother pushes my stroller past variegated crocus and palms reaching over the trailer park's crushed coquina road, the small tires lazily crunching the shell with each roll. We always stop at the common bathrooms housed in whitewashed stucco with green stains creeping up the outside.

At our trailer, chameleons scurry across the screens of the porch my father built as our living room. My mother, who grew up in the same South Philadelphia neighborhood as my father, puts me in my playpen wearing just a diaper because what could be better for a young child than fresh Florida air?

II. It could be anytime during my childhood. My bare chest presses against the cold x-ray plate. "Hold your breath," the cheerful technician says. The familiar whirring sound begins and stops. "Breathe." I exhale. "Good girl." She comes out of the booth and clanks the film plate out of its holder and clanks in another.

I am always a good girl. Even if it is one of those x-rays when I have to gag down chalky goo to light up my insides, I stand straight and stretch my arms long around the plate, never moving during that held breath. Every six months, the Doctors, the Interns, the Residents, the Nurses come to listen to my heart with their flat metal disks—a murmur, they had said at three months, hidden in the depths. Sometimes they attach wires that cling to my small body like a praying mantis, the suction cups the insect's delicate feet.

"A hole between the auricles," they teach me to say. How lucky I am to be living in this era with new discoveries every year, they say; children before weren't so lucky. My mother believes in technology and doctors; after all, my father is a rocket engineer. They will discover a way to fix my small heart, she is sure, just like they are sending men into outer space. We are not afraid.

And so my childhood is one of drawn blood, questions, and tests until the day a surgery is invented to fix me. In the meantime, I imagine that murmur as tiny lapping waves cooing over dark, wet sand.

III. A full-size cement dolphin at the entrance to the Sands Motel rises out of the waves, the spotlight at night making shadows on the cement foam. The ceaseless sound of surf surrounds us. In the years after the *Bumper* launch, my family, now with a little brother, moves to Brevard County, home to Cape Canaveral. Just about everyone here is from someplace else. The county population grows three hundred and seventy-five percent. I celebrate my eighth birthday here at the Sands as we wait for our cement-block "ranch" house to be built in the new subdivision.

My town of Satellite Beach is incorporated in 1957 after Percy Hedgecock and his brothers, Shine and Hub, begin developing their newly purchased hundred and thirty acres of saw palmetto and oak scrub. The land is "wild, raw, and unimproved," as the legal description reads. A giant metal balloon in the shape and features of a satellite is erected on the town's main road, State Road A1A running south to Sebastian Inlet.

Building and construction are a way of life as bulldozers destroy palmettos to make way for housing developments, shopping plazas, schools, and new businesses. Ditching and draining by big machinery continue day and night, turning wetlands into dry land for development. Mosquitoes are conquered with DDT, at least partially. The county population doubles again in the Sixties and Satellite Beach adopts the slogan "Where Progress Prevails."

An evangelical faith in technology and its role in creating good for all mankind sweeps down the beach. The space industry will prove our superiority to the atheistic Soviets, as all America knows, and should we flag in our efforts or will, the *beep-beep-beep* of Sputnik passing overhead every ninety-eight minutes spurs us on. The whole world is watching us and our little strip of sand. We see ourselves and our rockets on the TV news, in *Life* magazine, in newsreels before movies. The country is counting on us, all the families involved with the space industry, and no one is looking back. A newspaper photo shows the King and Queen of Belgium among the crowd at a launch, everyone wearing sunglasses, a few shielding their eyes from the glare, and all looking in exactly the same direction—up.

IV. My bedroom is still dark when my mother wakes me. "Time to get up, honey," she says. "Mmph," I grunt and pull the sticky sheet above my head. Outside my window insects, night birds I don't know the names for, armadillos, and gnawing, nibbling things click and scratch sporadically as they finish their nightly wandering.

"Remember how we are going to the beach to see Alan Shepard's rocket take off?" my mother nudges me. At the word "beach," my eyes open.

My six-year-old brother is already bounding into my room.

"Come on," he says. "We don't want to miss it."

"Get out of my room," I growl in my best ten-year-old sister voice.

In the dark morning, the kitchen and dining room are lit like a stage set waiting for us to prepare for our secret mission. We're going on an adventure, my sleep-fuzzy mind starts to realize as my mother puts bowls of Rice Krispies in front of my brother and me. My mother already has the radio on, and sure enough, the announcer tells us, importantly, "Today, May 5, 1961, we are going into space with Alan B. Shepard."

"He's scheduled to take off very early," my mother tells us, "but Daddy says there are always holds in the countdown, so we might have to wait for a while."

Daddy is already out at Cape Canaveral. When the countdowns get to a certain point, as everyone in school knows, the engineers are locked into the launch blockhouse for security and the flight coordinators, like my father, stay at their stations at Mission Control a couple miles away. My brother Ricky, my mother, and I will be going to Cocoa Beach to watch the launch, driving down onto the hard-packed sand and finding a good place to park. My mother has already filled the small aluminum cooler with sodas and bologna sandwiches.

They've closed school for the day so we can all watch this historic event. We have lots of historic events, living near Cape Canaveral. Alan Shepard will be the first American in space, flying *Freedom 7*. There are five Lindas in my class and we can all recite the names of the *Mercury 7* Astronauts. We call them out as we jump rope: "Car-penter, Coo-per, Glenn, and Grissom. Schir-ra, Shepard, and Mis-ter Slayton."

I pull on my two-piece bathing suit, then a clean shorts-set over it, the pink seersucker one with matching rickrack on the bottom of the legs and blouse, the one my mother finished just last week. Even though it's a warm May morning, the mugginess makes me a little cold and I put on my father's nylon windbreaker. It smells like Old Spice and cigarettes. My mother turns the lights off as we leave the house. The fronds on our palm trees hang slack in the stillness. Bright stars dot the blue-black sky.

V. A few months later, we are at the children's heart clinic in Miami where the catheterization is to take place. I walk in as if taking the stage for one of my dance recitals. We always come to this string of wooden World War II Army hospital buildings for checkups, and I know well the sound of our footfalls on the unpainted floorboards as we move from exam room to exam room. There is no air conditioning here, but the stethoscopes always feel cool and friendly on my chest.

For this event, I know a tube is going to be inserted into the vein in my right arm, the good vein, so perfectly visible at the right spot in the crease for blood tests. They'll put me under so I'll be asleep as they snake the tube up my vein, through the artery, and down into my heart. There the doctors will learn something new.

The grownups say this is the most important test yet. I get the feeling that what happens next depends on this one. I've overheard heard someone say, "this year," and maybe I also heard, "before it's too late." It seems like this is the beginning of a countdown.

VI. "Pre-teens," they call us, and we are on a church youth group "hayride" in the back of a pick-up truck with a couple bales of hay. We bounce south along the narrow patchwork stretch of A1A, getting farther and farther from what we know as civilization and our ordinary lives. Mile after mile of scrubby, gray-green palmettos pass. Beyond the narrow beam of the headlights, the scrub now seems interesting and mysterious, maybe a bit dangerous. We know snakes and raccoons ramble in there, maybe even panthers or bad men, but we speed past them all in our innocent confidence.

We have a mission tonight, a reason to be here during the full moon in May. This stretch of beach beyond the Eau Gallie Causeway and before the road ends at Sebastian Inlet is just sand, twenty miles of sand and waves that carry on seemingly forever, still wild enough that turtles come ashore this time of year to lay their eggs. We are silly pre-adolescents focused mostly on ourselves, the children of Cape Canaveral who have gone to the beaches a boring number of times to watch missile launches—but this time we are going to witness a natural event that has been going on for millennia.

South of Satellite Beach, the tiny towns thin out until the only lights on the side of the road are occasional motels built in the Fifties or even the Thirties. Appearing first is the warm glow above the palmettos, then the simple bulb illuminating a wooden or cement sign—the Surf Caster, the Dolphin, the Sea Turtle—and then the warm glow we leave behind.

VII. On the way to Shepard's launch, I get to sit in the front seat of the big Chevrolet, of course, because I'm older. Our car creeps down silent First Street, the headlights pointing east toward A1A. A tiny sliver of pink lies across the horizon as we turn onto the main road. A few other cars are on A1A, all heading in the same direction. My mother sits quietly, lit by the dashboard light, and even I don't feel like talking this early. My brother sucks his thumb in the dark back seat. The car engine hums the way cars seem to hum at night.

This part of A1A is maybe ten feet above beach level so that in the brightening light on the right side of the road I can look over the tops of the palmetto scrub to the ocean spreading all the way to Africa. The small morning waves roll languidly toward the shore; they have no place else to go. The beach is deserted, and the rise of palmettos above it stretch consistently the same height and density for miles.

The sun suddenly pops its orange edge above the horizon, and by the time we enter the outskirts of Cocoa Beach, the whole big ball floats on the water. *Maybe someday we'll go to the sun*, I think. After the moon, of course, as President Kennedy wants us to do this decade. My mother turns off the headlights and clicks on the radio. The only thing on either of the local AM stations is the launch.

My brother rouses in the back seat. "Are we there yet? When do we get to eat the sandwiches?"

Eventually we turn right and drive down the ramp to the beach, following the other cars. My mother finds a place to park and starts to back in like my father taught her. A fat man from the next car over with New Jersey license plates stands behind us to direct her to stop just before the wheels hit the soft part of the sand.

We climb out of the car and my mother gets out the beach blanket and spreads it on the roof. She puts the transistor radio on there, too, and turns it on. A commercial for Ipana toothpaste plays. My mother says the commercial must mean there's a hold in the countdown. Ricky opens the cooler and pulls out the bag of Fritos Corn Chips. "Can I open these?" he asks.

"Later," she says. "Get out your sand toys."

"I don't want to play," he says. "I wanna see the rocket."

He and I climb onto the car hood and scramble to the roof. There are hundreds, maybe thousands, of cars, pickup trucks, and even camper trailers parked on the sand, their front grills pointed toward the surf. It's more people than on a Sunday afternoon, and it's only seven o'clock on what would be a school day.

I strip down to my bathing suit, then head for the water, watching for the traffic still coming down. The wet sand is cold from the night and the water chills me as I wade out. It's almost flat calm, just small currents of waves rolling in. The sun, still low in the sky, is as white as if it has been up for hours, and a long ray of water sparkles under it, reaching from the horizon to the shore.

After swimming and floating, and making a sandcastle and moat, and climbing on and off the car roof, and not finding any kids I know, and talking to the very white, wrinkly Northerners who ask the question they always ask each other—where are you from?—and eating corn chips, I'm bored. My mother is comparing notes on the Jersey shore with our next-car neighbors.

"When are they going to shoot the rocket off?" Ricky asks.

"Can I walk down the beach to that place that sells tourist stuff?" I ask.

"Why didn't you bring a book?" my mother asks.

"Why didn't you remind me?"

"Can we get a hot dog?"

"It's almost two minutes!" shouts the fat man.

VIII. We turtle watchers finally pull over to a wide sandy patch and get out. Following a narrow path through the palmettos, we all know how to pick our way down to a beach. The lucky among us carry flashlights, and we turn them on to fleetingly light up patches of wilderness preserved like a jungle movie set, our beams crisscrossing. Anything could be lurking in the palmettos. The fronds clatter noisily against each other in the breeze.

The narrow path requires single file, and the noisy voices stretch out along the way. Sometimes a squeal rises up from one of us, something about stepping on sticker burrs or being brushed by the rough frond of a palmetto. The rising moon sits enticingly on the edge of the water, and the familiar surf urges us on. The beach ahead and the sandy path glow white. One by one, flashlights click off and voices quiet. We jump off the low edge of the dune and run through cold dry sand to wet sand and the lick of water.

I doubt any of us have seen a sea turtle before, except in an aquarium. Do the chaperones even know what to expect? But anything is possible in our era; we live with magic and mystery all the time. Rockets defy gravity, but prehistoric beasts ripe with eggs still climb out of the waves on a beach little changed from the days of the Ais Indians. On humid nights, we sit around our black-and-white televisions, insects crashing into the window screens, while reptiles creep up the beach under the moonlight. We giggle about boys at the edges of gymnasium sock hops as the cycle of life quietly turns elsewhere in the night.

Growing up in the go-go era of the Space Coast Sixties, we expect no less. We know we're going to defy gravity someday ourselves.

IX. Stretched out across her chenille bedspread, my mother and I are having a chat. We have never done this before, even though at age eleven there are some female things I probably need to know about. But it is not that kind of talk. Last night, as I was putting the dishes away, I told her I knew I was having an operation soon because I'd overheard her telling Grandmom, so my mother has decided to set up this talk about open-heart surgery.

She has spread out on the bed diagrams of hearts, the insides of them on graph paper, different angles with arteries cut short, and pictures of the operating room and machines. We talk of chambers and auricles and ventricles and the recently invented heart-lung machine that is making it all possible at this point in history. She shows me the picture in *Life* magazine with the machine and the tubes stretching from it. They disappear under the sheet covering the body on the table surrounded by masked and gowned surgeons.

I understand. I heard Mrs. Moxham from down the street tell my mother I am just too young to know what to expect. But I know what to expect. It's science, and I do well in science. I like having this important information that no one else at school has. I like having this very special heart problem.

But at this point, I don't know that the heart-lung machine has only been around a few years and has been used on just a handful of children. I don't know about the dogs and the chimps in the early surgeries. How some bled out during their operations. How some were poisoned by the wrong kind of blood, and how there might have been severe infections later for others. I don't know that surgeons need to experiment to learn how to do open-heart surgery, how most of the successful ones so far have all been closed heart. But to really fix things, like, say, a hole between the auricles, they need to cut open the heart.

I understand scientific experiments. That's what we need to do to get into space. Sometimes they don't work, I know. Sometimes the rockets blow up right on the launch pad or just fall over. Or they go off course, and the people in the blockhouse blow them up on purpose. Or they lose thrust and fall into the ocean.

Eventually, scientists feel good enough about what they learn to try it with humans. That's how they did it at the Cape— monkeys with wires and tubes clinging to their small bodies, then humans in space suits. Grownup hearts, then children's. Some don't get any worse. One or two get better. Some die. Do Mommy and Daddy know that?

X. My mother turns the transistor radio back on, which she had turned off to save the battery. We hear the announcer say it is two minutes and counting until liftoff. He tells us that Shepard will be able to talk to the control booth by space radio. Even my mother climbs onto the roof with us, holding our radio.

"One minute, thirty seconds to blastoff," the announcer says in his flat countdown voice. "The Redstone rocket carrying Alan Shepard into space is venting its liquid oxygen," he drones. We can't see any of this, of course, since we're almost ten miles away, just the flat-faced south shore of the Cape with a couple things sticking up out of it.

"Sixty seconds and counting," he notes. "Fifty seconds and counting."

My brother and I huddle close to our mother. The sounds of hundreds of radios all tuned to the same station drift up to us. The waves lap noiselessly against the sand.

"We're in the final stages of the countdown now," the announcer's voice rises just a little. "There goes the umbilical cord connecting the rocket to the rest of the world."

"T-minus ten," says the announcer. "Nine, eight, seven..."

"SIX, FIVE, FOUR, THREE, TWO, ONE," everyone on the shore shouts with the announcer, whose voice never changes.

"Zero," the announcer says. "Ignition. We can see the ignition. The rocket is beginning to rise, agonizingly slowly. And here we go. We are going into space with Alan B. Shepard," he declares. "It's rising slowly, painfully slowly. It looks so lonesome with that little red spotlight on the tail."

"There it is!" Ricky shouts simultaneously with thousands of other people on the beach. We all point toward a big, white-light ball followed by a long, fuzzy tail of smoke, some of it pink from the sun. The Redstone emerges from the top. "There it is! There it is," my brother says. The sun suddenly flashes off the missile's white side and everyone on the beach "ooohs."

The announcer follows the track of the rocket as if it were a horse race: "At T-plus thirty seconds, he's at five miles altitude. The first report from his microphone has just come in.

"He's twelve miles offshore now, outside the range of land-based rescue teams, over a string of search-and-rescue boats supplied by the Navy," the announcer informs us. An extra-bright, long, fiery, flash spurts from the bottom of the rocket and a burning chunk falls away. We've been trained to know that this is the rocket's first stage, which has used all its fuel, falling off and making its way down to the bottom of the ocean to join the debris of other rockets and the treasures of Spanish galleons.

The *Freedom 7* arcs down range toward the Bahamas and disappears into the atmosphere. Thousands of arms shield eyes against the sun like a mass salute. We all rotate south like radar domes watching the sky where the missile could be, far beyond the sight of regular human eyes.

"T-plus two minutes," the announcer continues. "He's a busy boy up there now. At thirty-three hundred miles per hour, Alan Shepard is the world's fastest man. T-plus two and a half minutes at forty miles altitude. The world's fastest traveling man. The engine's burned its fuel. He's almost weightless now.

"Ninety miles altitude!" the announcer shouts. "Alan Shepard is officially America's first man in space."

"Where is it, Mommy?" Ricky asks as we all stare at the perfectly blue sky.

"It's there," I say, watching the forever blue. "It's there."

XI. In the weeks before the surgery, I am not sleeping. My mother tells the doctors and everyone attributes it to the coming event. I am given tranquilizers and have a bad reaction, a hysterical one, thrashing and crying in my lavender bedroom.

My father comes in and sits on the side of my bed. I smell the ice cream on his breath, which is what he eats at night when he's trying to stay home and sober, making trip after trip to the refrigerator, the gentle opening and closing clicks of the freezer door like a lullaby. He strokes my sweaty forehead.

"I'm sorry to be so much trouble to everyone," I sob. "I'm sorry I have to have this operation, and Ricky has to stay at the Taylors' while we're away. And my kitty will be all alone—outside."

"You don't have anything to be sorry for," my father says. "It's not your fault. You'll be all better soon, and then I'll teach you how to do my special body flip into the waves."

"You already taught me that," I sniff.

"I know."

"Will you make sure the garage door is left up high enough for Bennie to get under?" I ask.

"Uh huh. I know just how high to make it. Bennie will be fine."

I start crying again. I don't cry much anymore, but I can't seem to help it now. I can't help thinking about Ricky and Bennie and Mommy and Daddy.

"I'm so sorry," I bawl again. "I'm sorry to be keeping you home at night so you can't go to the bar."

My father holds his breath for a second. "I want to be here," he says quietly. "I'd rather be here than at the bar. I want to be here with you and Mommy and Ricky."

"And Bennie," I sob.

"And Bennie."

XII. In the children's ward the night before the surgery, I think it doesn't look too bad because kids get to go up and down the hall in wheelchairs. I say "hi," and they say "hi" back. Mommy and Daddy and Grandmom and Grandpa Joe walk me to my room, and a nurse follows us in. My mother carries my little suitcase with my pajamas and some new books. Doctors, Residents, Interns, Nurses come in to listen to my heart. "They want to make sure it's still there before they operate," my father jokes.

They tell me how they will put the mask over my face. How I should just breathe normally, and the funny smelling gas will make me go to sleep. How the heart-lung machine will do my breathing and heartbeat for me so I can be very, very still for the doctors. How when I wake up, my heart will be fixed.

How they will put the mask over my face, and I should just breathe normally, and the funny smelling gas will make me go to sleep. How the heart-lung machine will do my breathing and heartbeat for me so I can be very, very still for the doctors, and when I wake up, my heart will be fixed. How they will put the mask over my face how I should just breathe normally and the funny smelling gas will make me go to sleep how the heart-lung machine will do my breathing and heartbeat for me...

XIII. The beach world drops away—boys, girls, trucks, flashlights. I am alone with the sand and the night around me. The moon, low on the horizon, sends a long ray of yellow across the surface of the water. The moon-baked waves run toward the shore, over and over, the white foam edge glowing, then cresting to fall in a delicate fringe murmuring up the dark wet sand. The sound surrounds the beach, fills the air, repeats itself like a chant.

Soon something unformed rises and falls with the waves, closer and closer, rises and falls—a tiny head, front flippers, the big shell gliding through the water—until one wave strands her and she begins her slow plod up the sand. Her great shell dips side to side as she makes her way above the high tide line. She finds her spot and starts to dig, thrashing and throwing a halo of sand, soft and bright with moonlight. She settles into her spot and drops her eggs one by one into the nest, her eyes dumb and unfocused. The moon climbs over the crest of the beach, hovers.

XIV. My mother waits and waits. The surgery plan is for four hours, but four hours, five, seven, nine pass while the OR nurses go in and out. My parents have already been informed that no one will be allowed to tell them anything until it's over. My father reads much more of *The Rise and Fall of the Third Reich* than he intended. Probably hanging on the wall is one of those plain white-faced clocks with big black hands and numbers that my parents don't want to look at. Beyond those wide swinging doors, I am sleeping.

Finally the surgeon emerges, shakes my father's hand. "Everything is fine," he says. "A bit more complicated than expected. But Linda is fine."

It's then he tells them for the first time the story he will have to repeat later so they can take it all in, a story that wasn't in the diagrams on my mother's bed: *There wasn't just the hole . . . we found more than expected . . . three veins on the wrong side of the heart . . . had to medically freeze the brain for thirty minutes, life processes stopped . . . a piece of Teflon tubing through the hole to plug it and drain the veins into the right side . . . there permanently . . . should be no problem, should work . . . the Teflon? . . . yes, the same thing they use in astronaut suits . . . no, it's not usual.*

XV. Hours later, the turtle scatters loose sand into a fine, thick cover for the eggs, and without looking back, makes her way again into the indifferent water.

COWBOYS

Science is an endless frontier.
–Heart Surgeon Walt Lillehei

Sitting on the floor in front of our TV and wearing my cowgirl outfit, I saw Fess Parker (playing Davy Crockett) as all man—strong but gentle, firm but kind. After all, he "killed him a ba'r when he was only three," as the show's theme song told us. Every week, I sang along: "Davy, Davy Crockett. King of the wild frontier." He lived out in the wilds because he wanted to do things his way without the confines of life "back East."

Maybe it was the buckskin, the fringe hanging off his wide shoulders and moving in rhythm with his long stride. I could imagine how it smelled—like my father's suede jacket. Or maybe it was the way Davy so casually carried his rifle, as if it were nothing, really. Everyone else on the show listened to what he had to say, a take-charge kind of guy. I liked the way he sometimes wore the fluffy tail of his coonskin cap coming forward over his shoulder, like a beauty queen's lock of hair. And I especially liked the way he squinted under that cap. He was cool, before I even knew there was such a thing as cool.

Frontiersmen were everywhere on TV in those days, morphing from a Kentucky backwoodsman like Davy to trail-riding cowboys to dubious "lawmen." Maverick, Matt Dillon, Ben Cartwright and his boys—every night of the week, there were cowboys on TV. A certain amount of righteousness surrounded them all, an attitude of being able to take care of anything, and—most importantly—a going-it-alone, renegade style. We trusted cowboys, even though they were gamblers. After all, they helped open up the American West.

It's hard for people today to appreciate what it was like at a time when nobody knew what would happen when, for example, when you stuck a needle into a heart.

–Surgeon Henry Swan, one of the first to use induced hypothermia in open heart surgery

Paladin, the lead character of the show *Have Gun, Will Travel*, rode into my consciousness on his black horse. The deep vocals of the program's theme song told us: "Have gun, will travel is the card of a man. A knight without armor in a savage land." It was the Sixties by then, and Paladin was even more independent than Davy. Paladin was a paid assassin—an outlaw, really. He dressed all in black, refined and classy, always wearing a narrow black cowboy tie. He squinted, too, under a black hat. The black holster low on his slim hips was embossed with a silver chess knight, like the knights on my father's chessboard.

> *There were virtually no*
> *regulations to hold them back.*
> –David K. C. Cooper in *Open Heart:*
> *The Radical Surgeons Who Revolutionized Medicine*

The Space Coast I grew up on was the new Wild West, with palmettos rather than sagebrush. President Kennedy called it "the Next Frontier." For cowboys, we had astronauts—test pilots who had cut their eyeteeth by joyriding in expensive jets. Sometimes they got into trouble, crash landing wherever they could find a spot and miraculously walking away; other times they had to bail out and let the plane go on without them.

Legends of the astronauts' shenanigans circulated through the press. Tom Wolfe immortalized it all in his nonfiction novel *The Right Stuff*—the wild parties at the Holiday Inn, the bikinis on Canaveral pier, the pioneering topless bars, and the free Corvettes provided to the astronauts every year by the enterprising Chevy dealer Jim Rathman, cars the astronauts used to drag race down the main street of Cocoa Beach.

The young rocket engineers, like my father, already had a reputation for hard partying from their GI Bill college days. There were plenty of things to commemorate on the Space Coast. In the heady early days, tourists and locals alike ran into the streets yelling "Missile! Missile!" whenever there was one streaking through the atmosphere—or fizzling into disaster. The famous hot spot Bernard's Surf, my father's favorite watering hole, gave out free drinks if you were there when a missile went off. Even a disaster was an occasion for liquid solace.

Engineers involved in a particular launch were locked into the launch blockhouse at a certain point in the countdown for safety and to foil Soviet spies, which we imagined might be hanging around. Whether the shot was successful or "scrubbed," once released, the engineers headed into town like cowboys just off the trail.

I think we had a mortality of 35%.
–Surgeon Viking Bjork on using the heart-lung machine and induced hypothermia simultaneously

My father played out his cowboy persona with a .22 pistol the year we lived in Sunnyvale for his temporary job at the Satellite Test Center in California. Some Saturdays, he took my brother and me out to a gravel pit in the hills for target practice. I aimed for those concentric circles off in the distance, just like my father showed me. The kickback, relatively small, made my ten-year-old arm jump. My father knelt behind my brother, who was only six, to hold his arm up when it was his turn.

Afterwards we studied the little holes we'd made in the target paper, unable to tell whose was whose. We stood together in the faint autumn sunlight—Central California before the rains—with the smell of dry leaves, my father's suede jacket, and his Chesterfields all mixing together. It always hung around him, that outlaw smell, but he wasn't really an outlaw himself. He didn't have the heart of one.

It was that Thanksgiving out west when my father shot himself in the thigh practicing his "quick draw," like on *Gunsmoke*, Jim Beam by his side, my brother's toy plastic holster strapped to his leg. The women and kids were back at the house helping my aunt clean up dinner when my uncle brought him hobbling in, blood streaming down his leg.

They didn't bleed on television shows and we all stared in fascination. "He got me. He got me. The S.O.B. got me," my father, the great kidder, moaned in mock agony. My mother took him to the hospital where they pulled the bullet out and stitched him up.

One of his buddies later made him a commemorative wooden plaque—a two-foot-by-ten-inch piece of pine stained a dark brown and carved with the tribute: "Dick 'Quick Draw' Buckmaster. November 24, 1960." Mounted in the center like an antelope rack was the bullet.

Meet me at the airport in Denver.
You'll recognize me—I'll be
wearing a cowboy hat.
–Surgeon Henry Swan to David K. C. Cooper

You could recognize cowboys by their hats, surgeons by their scrubs, and the astronauts, when they were in town, by their big, shit-eating grins. These heroes were always the good guys, even if their methods were a bit unorthodox.

When my surgeon discovered something wrong, he quickly decided to induce hypothermia. Three errant veins were carrying blood to the wrong side of my heart. Rather than circulating through my body, the blood was circling round and round my heart. In my imagination, I see him suddenly seize a piece of Teflon tubing hanging in the operating room. He threaded the tube into the veins, then through the hole in my heart, and solved both problems in the process by plugging the hole and draining the veins on the right side. This had never been done before. It was an improvised solution, new medical territory. It was a maverick move.

TECHNICALLY

I. On May 4, 1962, I was technically dead, they tell me. They had cooled my brain during the surgery, frozen it so it couldn't interfere with procedures in my chest, and I was not alive. Just like that, they say, "You were technically dead for thirty minutes."

"Linda was technically dead for thirty minutes," my parents tell my grandparents, the neighbors, and the newspaper reporter who does a story on me as the American Heart Association poster child for the county spring fundraising drive. They all look at me as if my parents had said, "Linda just learned to ride her bike without training wheels."

I was technically dead for thirty minutes: No thinking in that state, no wondering, no thoughtless impulse even. Just being. Or not being. Only silence, perhaps, like deep space, a trillion stars staring eyelessly. No gravity, just hovering, maybe, above the crowd around the table, as if to decide whether to continue toward that farther light or to return to the small, cold body.

I never got to make that choice, technically. They made it for me and brought me back, like Mission Control brought Alan Shepard back from outer space one year earlier, almost to the day. We were both miracles of science, though technically perhaps, there are no such things as miracles.

II. Atrial septal defect and anomalous pulmonary venous return, congenital heart disease present at birth, technically.

III. From the BBC article: "Surgeons Use Cold to Suspend Life":

"The patients undergo induced hypothermia. Their body is cooled from its normal temperature of 37C (98.6F) to just 18C (64.4F). Dr. John Elefteriades explains, 'The body is essentially in true, real-life, suspended animation, with no pulse, no blood pressure, no signs of brain activity. The patient is indistinguishable from someone who is actually dead. The technique of extreme cooling is fascinating. It takes the moment of death and smears it out.'"

IV. Also left behind, unknowingly, like a small surgical sponge, was an ambivalence, a hesitation, a tiny bit of frozen matter. I never got to make that choice, technically—farther light or small cold body?

V. Through the miracle of Teflon, my mother can fry an egg without it sticking to the pan.

Through the miracle of Teflon, the astronauts won't get burned up in their space suits.

Through the miracle of Teflon, they plug the hole in my heart and drain the misplaced veins into the right side.

VI. No big deal. "I was technically dead for thirty minutes," I said repeatedly for years.

I stopped saying it my junior year of high school.

As an adult, I would say it with an ironic laugh: "I was technically dead for thirty minutes."

VII. Is "technically dead" the same as "dead"?

If you come back, were you really "dead"?

Doesn't "dead" mean forever?

I remember when my cat Bennie died, it was like he was frozen stiff and didn't thaw.

What if the moment of death is "smeared out"?

I've read since then that people who have "near death" experiences see all kinds of amazing things. But of course, I wasn't *near* death; I was technically dead.

VIII. What else happened that year I was dead? John Glenn orbited the earth three times in his space capsule. Telstar, our first communication satellite, was launched into space (it's still out there). The first part of the summer was like suspended animation. I had to be very careful so the breastbone could grow back together. The doctors took the stitches out, all one hundred and four of them.

All the other girls in the seventh-grade locker room wore bras, so my mother bought me a training bra even though I didn't need one. It covered the scar. (I heard my father tell her that psychologically it was the thing to do.) I got a haircut that was supposed to make me look like Hayley Mills in *The Parent Trap*, but it didn't. I went to a party and danced with a boy. Technically, I became a teenager.

HEIDI

Walking home from Sea Park Elementary, I am sticky and sweaty under my cotton dress, and my red bookbag swings at my side. I imagine I'm climbing through fields of willowy grasses and alpine wildflowers, butterflies leading the way, goats daintily leaping from rock to rock, and little birds singing in the thicket, whatever a thicket is. I am Heidi now, from the book about the girl in Switzerland. Like her, I am barefoot, carrying my clunky buckle school shoes.

A dense shadow of dark green Christmas trees lines the field. The sun in my story, a pale yellow, is soft and warm, the air crisp. Soon I will be high enough into the mountains to get to the part with the snow, which I will cheerfully skip through, as if it is a field of cold cotton balls that give way under my feet. It's possible a big blizzard will roll through, blinding my way and wrapping me in the most freezing blanket I can imagine. This will be dangerous, but do-able—a certain cold thrill with a touch of suffering and lots of fortitude—and I will be just like the pioneer women on the TV shows.

Gone is the flat, asphalt street baking under the Florida sun, a street with no shady spots because there are no shrubs or trees, only young palmetto palms—two to a yard—planted as the last step in the creation of our new subdivision. The rough lawns no longer run ragged along the edge of the asphalt in the late afternoon humidity. As long as I am Heidi, I'm not returning to our flat cement block ranch-style house on Albatross Drive, empty until my little brother arrives home from Mrs. Aston's kindergarten and my mother from her job as a secretary at the bank shortly thereafter, and maybe—eventually—my father.

Instead, I'm on my way to Grandfather's hut with the pointy roof made of real wood from trees. Rather than getting myself a peanut butter on toast sandwich with a Coke, Grandfather will hand me a bowl of warm milk fresh from the cow, or maybe from a goat, although I don't know how you get milk from a goat. At Grandfather's I won't be settling in with my latest Weekly Reader Book of the Month Club story but will instead climb a ladder upstairs to sleep in the hayloft.

The story of Heidi takes place in the "olden days." I love the olden days. Grandfather lives a life just like the old New Englanders way up north in the Nineteenth Century. His farm implements, the few that he has, are hand-made of wood or basic metal. The little stool that I sit upon is the same kind of stool I've seen in fairy tales that peasants sat upon centuries before. Life in the mountains is simple—no rockets, no doctors or hospitals, no waiting for Daddy to come home. In the mountains, Heidi runs free.

ONLY NINETY MILES AWAY

I was twelve in October 1962, at the outbreak of the Cuban Missile Crisis. The only thing I knew about Communist Cuba was the hand-drafted diagram released by the CIA showing the small island. Published relentlessly in the *Orlando Sentinel* and in my father's weekly *Time* magazine, and shown in close-up on our television screen by Huntley and Brinkley, the diagram was pimpled with tiny location markers for surface-to-air missile (SAM) launch pads, Cruise missile sites, airfields, and medium-range ballistic missiles (MRBM). And just north of the island, across only ninety miles of bright turquoise water, was the tip of our very own state, the string of Florida Keys where we snorkeled on family vacations, now sitting naked and exposed to the godless "Reds."

Only ninety miles away we heard, over and over, on the nightly news. President Kennedy told us in grave terms during a special television broadcast that "each of these medium-range missiles is capable of striking Washington, D.C., the Panama Canal, Cape Canaveral, or any other city in the southeastern part of the United States." *Cape Canaveral.* We were practically the bullseye in the diagram of the MRBM's range. *It could happen at any time.*

For my father, and everyone else's in our neighborhood, missiles were a daily topic of conversation in Satellite Beach. The U.S. had launched its own practice medium-range missiles from the Cape starting in the 1950s, so our fathers knew what they were capable of doing.

The reality in Cuba was stark in the photographs brought back by the U-2 spy plane. We kids had never seen photos from so high up, and the clear resolution of the tiny trees and thin roads winding to the toy-sized buildings made it all real—real trees, real buildings hiding real missiles. There were even tents in the photo, *where Russian soldiers could be sleeping only 90 miles away.*

"It was a shame we never got to Cuba," one of my parents would occasionally say. What they meant was they had never gone for a weekend of nightclub hopping, cheap rum, cigars (even if you didn't smoke cigars), and wild Latin rumba *before*—before the Revolution under Fidel Castro in 1959. This exotica, only a boat ride from our shores, had even more palm trees, bougainvillea, and lizards than the tiny, tropical trailer park where my grandmother lived in Miami on Southwest Eighth Street, the same trailer park where I started life in 1950 while my father studied at the University of Miami.

My parents grew up as city people in South Philadelphia and liked nightlife. In the early Fifties, Miami was the place for it: the Beachcomber with its faux South Seas décor, the Latin Quarter, Vagabond's, strip joints like The Jungle. Most of those places were out of reach for my parents, who were living on the GI Bill and my father's part-time lifeguard job at Matheson Hammock. That didn't keep them at the trailer park though, and my mother's mother would walk down from her trailer to babysit me once a week. Even at the cheaper clubs—dives catering to ex-GIs and their dates—they could hear the latest Latin music and watch saucy women dance in costumes skimpier than the bathing suits on Miami Beach.

When my father eventually moved us north to the Cape Canaveral area, my grandmother "Mamie" (the derivation on "Mary" she picked up during the war when she worked as a riveter at the Navy Yard) continued to live in the same trailer park. During our childhood visits with my mother to Grandmom's, my little brother and I slept on the screened porch that doubled as the living room for her trailer. On the wood paneling curved to the back wall of the trailer ran a little rail where Grandmom displayed the blown glass knickknacks she collected. She would let me rearrange them on the railing if I was careful. I held each one up to the window—the ballerina, the giraffe—and the semitropical light made them glow.

Into her sixties, my grandmother worked as a "salesgirl" in the venerable Hartley's Department Store downtown. Our visits usually included a trip to Hartley's to visit Grandmom at work so she could show us off to her co-workers and show us her luxurious workplace, where she wasn't allowed to take time off to talk to us. She would pretend to be re-folding the blouses while we stood close by, jabbering away. The three of us had taken the local bus in—a thrill to us car-dependent Space Coast suburbanites with nothing urban in our vicinity—and walked from the stop to the store, just like Grandmom did every day. Grandmom, who didn't drive, knew city bus schedules and routes like some people knew the Miami Jockey Club horse racing sheets. She could get us anywhere.

By the early Sixties, we were walking past the "Se Habla Español" signs in the storefronts, something that would always draw a "tsk tsk" from my grandmother. Hartley's didn't have such signs in their windows, as least not yet. Wealthy women from Cuba and Central and South America had always flown in to Miami for weekend shopping sprees in stores like Hartley's and Burdine's, but these newcomers were different; as far as my grandmother was concerned, they didn't have the money.

Little Havana sprang up almost overnight after the first nine Cuban escapees were rescued by the Coast Guard from a tiny boat off the Dry Tortugas in 1959. The earliest wave was immigrants with political connections, supporters of Batista escaping Castro's new government. A few scattered Cuban pastry and coffee shops opened, and late at night a couple of Miami radio stations played two or three hours of Cuban music.

The next arrivals were wealthy landowners and professionals. Everyone, Cubans and Americans alike, thought the new residents were just temporary, that the Castro government would never last, that we'd never allow a Communist dictator so close to the United States. We Floridians cheered and wept as the planeloads of children arrived during Operation Pedro Pan, innocent children airlifted from the clutches of Fidel Castro. We hated the Communists on the island, not the freedom seekers who were arriving and were quickly processed by immigration.

As time went on, the immigrants' wealth back home was nationalized, and small merchants and skilled laborers fled the island. The dark knowledge that they may never leave settled over South Florida and the refugee community. By 1962, eighteen hundred Cubans were landing in Miami every week. Reluctantly, the immigrants found they needed to turn to the

U.S. and Dade County governments for financial assistance, and even more reluctantly, the governments distributed it.

To white Miamians like my grandmother, it seemed as if loud Latin music had invaded the downtown streets. It was all right to go to nightclubs to hear such music and watch scantily clad Latinas dance, but the daytime downtown was for business and middle-class white women shoppers. Cuban men in starched white guayaberas were now playing dominoes at street-side tables and sipping from tiny cups of strong coffee. "Why aren't they working," my grandmother would sniff.

Women with voluminous black hair in tight dresses and pedal pushers strolled by in "mules," confidently mincing on the spikes of those backless pumps with the hip swing that the shoes encouraged. Women in Hartley's didn't dress like this. As I watched these women pass, I noticed how their bare brown heels were rough and cracked over the edges of the shoes. Everyone in Florida had rough, cracked heels from going barefoot or wearing sandals all the time, but these feet were different from mine—these were foreign heels.

Almost no Cubans lived on our stretch of peninsula along the Space Coast; the "immigrants" there were people like us, the families of educated engineers who came to work at the Cape. But everywhere in South Florida, whites complained about the street behavior of "the Cubans." "Why can't they speak English," was the common refrain we heard from my grandmother and every other white person we met down there.

Grandmom should have been no stranger to a community living loudly on the street. Both sides of my family were from the rough and tumble streets of South Philly, the kind of neighborhood where mothers bellowed off the front porches for Joey or Julio to come home, and other mothers bellowed back, "He's over here!" or "They went down to the dump to ice skate!" My father's mother, Grandmom Buck, could sit in the swing on her front porch and hold a conversation with Mrs. Concello sitting on the next porch over, who could gossip in Italian with the neighbor on the other side of her.

As a child, I didn't really understand how Cubans living in Miami was a different situation, except that here it was foreign voices and browner people. Resentment of the freedom seekers grew, and many Miamians nodded as television reporter Wayne Farris described them as "houseguests who have worn out their welcome. The Cubans are a threat to our businesses and our tourist economy."

Which was more of a threat, I wondered in my childish way, Cubans in Miami or Communists in Cuba? Although no one ever confused the two or suspected those in Miami to be Communists, it was confusing to believe everything the grownups said, at least until the missiles arrived. With their arrival, it was clear that Communists could actually land on our shores and invade our homes, taking away our American way of life. Castro himself might even come! I was afraid they would confiscate my bike for Communist kids. The only milk we would be allowed would be coconut milk and our regular milk would be sent to Russia, where everyone was starving. They would make us eat their terrible food, black beans. Whoever heard of *black* beans? They must be rotten, we surmised by their color, and we had learned there were tiny pebbles mixed in so we would break our teeth, our beautiful American teeth.

If refugees with only the clothes on their backs could traverse those *ninety miles* in small, leaking boats with failed engines, I reasoned, imagine what the Communists could do in powerful Soviet warships. The Red Threat hovered over our days. Every evening, the same pictures on TV showed Soviet ships steaming toward their comrades on that tiny, misled island. Every evening, newsreels ran footage of American ships headed toward Europe, where the Iron Curtain, which I imagined as a giant sheet of chainmail stretched across the continent, trapped people on the other side.

At school we rehearsed for annihilation, practicing "duck and cover" exercises when we tipped our desks over to face Cape Canaveral and knelt behind them to deflect the inevitable explosion from that most desirable target. And looming over our shoulders was Fidel—the beard, the cigar, the fatigues, the gesticulations. Watching the news with the families in our Florida rooms, our fathers spat out: *Castro.*

The only actual Cuban I knew the name of was Ricky Ricardo, Lucy's husband on the TV show. He had a real accent, but somehow it was okay that he was married to a white woman. We never questioned his friendship with those whitest of Americans, Fred and Ethel, and the fact that he lived in a regular middle-class apartment. Lucy got into lots of trouble, but being married to a Cuban wasn't one of them. Ricky even spoke Spanish on the show sometimes, as if it were perfectly normal, even though Lucy made fun of him. Maybe it was because he was an *entertainer*, a Latin orchestra leader in a nightclub where the audience sat at little round tables with cocktails in front of them, just as I imagined my parents had done on their nights out.

At the end of the weekly episode, Ricky performed a piece with his band, a big band with horns and saxophones and bongos and guitars, just like you would expect to see in a Havana club—but almost all the members of Ricky's band were white. Wearing shirts with giant ruffled sleeves, they flashed when they played. Ricky wore a modified tux and his conga hung across his chest from his shoulder. The music itself was modified *salsa* for American audiences and Cuban *son*, a mixture of Old World *cancion* and African rhythms with American big band flourishes and lots of television smiles. The band members always stood up in unison when things got fiery, and when Ricky really got going on his conga, his hair fell over his forehead and flew out of place in the back.

Ricky was a different man during these sets, not just the long-suffering husband he played on the show, the straight man for Lucy's shenanigans. There he would be—in front of the band, singing and dancing those mincing Cuban salsa steps. His slim hips and knees swung smoothly back and forth in time to the music as he made his way across the floor, sidling up to one of the tables to sing to the woman watching his every move. Sometimes he would wear a debonair little straw hat he would doff and place over his heart for the romantic parts. On stage, Ricky was in charge. It was his show.

My grandmother was something of a "Lucy" character herself, a bit of a ditz, a girl from a city neighborhood who put on airs, even as a salesgirl. She met Joe, who became her third husband, on New Year's Eve at the downtown VFW. Joe was an all-around good guy, everybody's friend, who managed the Cocktail Lounge a few doors down from Hartley's, the lounge not exactly a joint but an old-fashioned neighborhood bar where businessmen stopped by for a quick one after leaving the office. Joe had a special joke for everyone, depending on your interest, but I never heard him tell a Cuban joke. Nevertheless, despite its downtown location, the Cocktail wasn't a place a Cuban would wander into, at least not while Joe was still there.

Joe adored my grandmother, his Lucy, and they bought a new "townhouse" in Hialeah as the Cuban neighborhood crept down Eighth Street. Joe did quite well at the Cocktail, better than you would think from the look of the fading booth banquettes and the rickety bar stools. Joe was a New York street boy, and there was some kind of arrangement with the Long Island owner. Every night after closing, from the large bar-sized bottles under the counter, Joe refilled the "nips," the miniature bottles that some of his customers returned in an era before returnables. Haig & Haig, Seagrams 7, Jim Beam, and of course, Bacardi rum were popular with those same customers, and none of them objected to the lack of a federal seal on the top of the bottle.

Miami had always been that kind of place. Rum mysteriously arrived during Prohibition. Money flowed in and out unnoticed. Land scams caused a big boom and bust during the Twenties. And any kind of "import" arrived on airstrips at the edge of the Everglades and at docks hidden in the mangroves of the Keys.

Most people forgot, if they ever knew, that during Prohibition more than booze arrived on our shores from Cuba. After the 1924 passage of immigration quotas for people from particular countries, there was a lucrative trade in illegal immigrants through Havana to South Florida; if Eastern and Southern Europeans or Chinese could get themselves to the island, they could easily find "charter" boats to take them over the water, where they would be dropped off on isolated beaches and in the mangroves. The charter boats guaranteed success; if the passengers got caught and sent back to Havana, they could get a free ride the next time.

It was okay for music from the Caribbean to arrive on our shores, or food, or rum, or bright colors, or even architectural styles—but poor people were always less welcome. Down at the end of that long peninsula jutting into the sea, so far from the rest of the Eastern Seaboard, Florida seemed to be just waiting for invaders.

Now with the Missile Crisis, the most dangerous things imaginable could strike our sandy, sunny shores at any time. Those missiles carrying atomic warheads, capable of arching over the curve of the earth, might smash into our homes without warning. It didn't matter if Satellite Beach was over two hundred miles from Key West—poor Key West, only ninety miles from Cuba—because that extra distance was nothing to a missile.

THE MOSQUITO TRUCK

Thick-headed fog roams street to street, engulfing kids in white clouds fuming from the back of the big truck. Down First, over Sea Gull, up Second, around all the numbered streets and past our house on Albatross Drive. Mosquitoes are the foe; the DDT spewing from the back of a truck is our big science. We believe in big science—that's how our daddies' rockets are going to beat the Russians.

The cloud billows and blooms dense and white. The boys on their bikes whoop and holler from inside the soft tunnel, following as the truck makes its rounds. The only thing visible is a wheel spoke here, a foot on a pedal there, a wild face squinting. Ghost boys appear and disappear behind a noisy ghost machine, following the call.

We girls hang back a bit on our bikes, where the fumes are thinner. We squeal. Our eyes burn. We're repulsed by the stench. But we, too, love the mystery of the fog; we want the magic of invisibility, the coy visibility. We want to be lost in a way you can't ever be lost under the blasting Florida sun.

The boys will eventually grow to up to be soldiers and disappear into the fog of jungle, or slide away into narcotic mists, or stalk the miasma of manhood. We girls hang back a bit. We want to believe in mystery. We want to believe we will fall in love and turn into princesses.

EVOLUTION

We are teenagers, just barely. It's summer—long, hot, sticky, stifling summer. Our tans are sunburned. My freckles run together. Flat-chested and long-torsoed, we wear bikinis. The high loop of my scar shows above my top. Marie has hips, but I'm narrow as an egret, not an elegant snowy egret, but a short, pencil-legged wader.

The beach is full of midges, invisible biters that like our salty skin, attacking from every direction. The air refuses to move. The tide is so far out that thin shelves of coquina lie exposed with weak tidal pools between. Offshore, the flat, tropical-gray sea is warm enough for sharks, but we see nothing on the tepid horizon. It beckons and we start toward it.

Soon, though, it's too much trouble to walk out to the water. Even our summer-tough feet can barely stand the coquina's rough surface, white hot under the afternoon sun. We step into a soft pool, silky sanded bottom, water just above our ankles.

We lie down on our backs, settling like sediment. The water is as warm as embryonic fluid. It almost covers out stomachs. Our hair floats like seagrass. The heartless sun scorches our salted skin.

We turn onto our stomachs and push on the sand back and forth, the water riding the backs of our legs. We are amoebas, primitive nummulites, plankton governed by currents and moon. We pose like ancient lizardfish balancing on pelvic fins just before they first walked ashore.

DESIRE

Latin music was the night music of my adolescence, alone in my bedroom with my red plastic transistor radio tuned to the Cuban stations out of Miami 200 miles away. I was only able to pick them up after dark, in those days before FM, the night air capturing transmissions unseen during the daytime. I turned the radio this way and that to grab what I could of those broadcasts in a language unknown to me, absorbing the rolls and rhythms of something I didn't understand. Stations faded in and out, snippets of music alternating with the static of distance and desire.

It wasn't all musical. Long segments of talk took up some of the programs. Of course I couldn't understand, but I could hear the anger and frustration and sadness in those voices. Once in a while I could make out the word *Castro*.

The bedroom door was always closed. The sticky Florida air hovered around my lavender room with matching bedspread and the bright red radio. I soaked up the tunes and counter-tunes that moved over, under and around, riding on horns, congas, guitars, marimbas, calling voices, predictable but always surprising. Shot through the music, no matter how upbeat, was an inexplicable longing, like that of a troubadour singing under the balcony of his beloved night after warm night, waiting for an appearance, hoping for an answer.

The music had everything I thought I needed and wanted—a layering of sounds and calling from someplace else. Music in exile, music that was packed up and brought along like the bits of old family silver and black-and-white photographs with palm trees in the background, music you had to take with you when you had to leave, as I knew I eventually would.

STAGE II: FALLOUT

The fact is, that people cannot come to heartily like Florida till they *accept* certain deficiencies as the necessary shadow to certain excellences.

-HARRIET BEECHER STOWE, *PALMETTO LEAVES*

High above the mast the moon
Rides clear of her mind and the waves make a refrain
Of this: that the snake has shed its skin upon
The floor.

-WALLACE STEVENS, "FAREWELL TO FLORIDA"

ON THE ROAD TO HOME

The girl was to drop me off in New London, to catch a ferry to the island. It was 1969, the summer after my first year of college, and I had landed a job waitressing at the country club on Fishers Island in Long Island Sound. Through a friend of a friend, I connected with her, a girl whose name I will never remember, who was driving back home in her red Karmann Ghia. We were all "girls" back then, veering either into motherhood, the typing pool, or becoming a "chick"—a newly liberated woman who was supposed to be equally comfortable with flower power and revolutionary politics.

I knew very little about "up North." To me, New England and New London sounded far away and exotic, and kind of foggy, like the olden days I'd read about in *The House of the Seven Gables*. I didn't know about ferries or summer seasons bookended by Memorial Day and Labor Day. I didn't know about old money and summer homes opened by caretakers. I didn't know there still were houses with wooden floors and third-floor dormers looking out on oak trees, where the hired girls like me were boarded. I thought such things only existed in the books I read lying on the terrazzo floor of our Florida room, shaded by a solitary palm.

What I did know, as the girl and I left my parents' house in Satellite Beach, was that Fishers Island was part of New York State and that the drinking age was eighteen there. I also knew that we—two chicks in a red Ghia, top down, short shorts and hippie hair turning north onto A1A—looked really good.

Why should the boys have all the fun, I wondered in high school. Kerouac, Kesey, Ginsberg, Snyder, Thoreau, and before them, the men of English literature class—Byron, Whitman, Wordsworth. Our surfer boyfriends would pack up their boards and fly to Eleuthera in the Bahamas in search of the perfect wave; the ones who had saved more money from their summer jobs could go to Southern California and slip over the border for underage beer. Why not me, I thought, why not us? Young white women in the 1960s with the Pill and driver's licenses, we could go on the road, too.

After all, we were Americans, and it was our birthright. Packing up and taking off just for the hell of it was in our chromosomes. Rock and roll and the literature of the Beats spawned the restlessness of hippies, and although I couldn't find the character that was "me" in the tales of male adventures, I knew the itch that floated from the pages of books and acid rock airwaves.

The men in those books, boozers or dopers though they might have been, were cool, despite the pain they might have caused others flying by as the wheels ate up the miles. I bought it all. I wanted to go with them—across the country, hopping a steamer to the Far East, slipping over the border to far out Mexico, hiking to a fire lookout with a pack full of books.

But most of all, I wanted to *be* them. I wanted to go whenever and wherever I wanted. Sure, there had been women on some of the trips in those books, even babies sometimes. But that wasn't the same. That wasn't doing it yourself, calling the shots. It wasn't *driving*.

Our mothers had learned to drive from their husbands so they could take us to dance classes and swimming pools and load the station wagon with groceries at the shopping center. They collected S&H Green Stamps to satisfy their desires for toasters and blenders. We, their daughters, were the first "drivers' ed" generation. Our passing the driving test was a rite of passage comparable to our mothers putting on their first pair of nylon stockings with a seam up the back, in the days before the war. That first class behind the wheel in the shopping center parking lot across from Satellite High was my ticket to everything my mother didn't have.

In the early days, before my brother was born, when it was just me and no car air conditioning, my parents drove all night through the Southwest to escape the heat of the day. It was the beginning of the aerospace industry, and my father followed the jobs around the country—Long Beach, Norfolk, Maryland, and later, Cape Canaveral.

It would have been some kind of Chevrolet coupe we were in, second-hand. That's what he always drove, and I still associate the rounded lines and grinning grills of the early 1950s models with the possibilities of family.

In the mornings, we would pull into a motel where I amused myself with books and dolls while they slept. My mother woke late morning and took me to the pool so my father, the driver, could get a few more hours sleep. After lunch in the car, he would tell jokes and sing loudly in what he called his "whiskey tenor." "When the moon hits the eye like a big pizza pie, that's *amore*," he sang, never finishing a whole song.

We drove through the afternoon and evening, the desert landscape rolling by. After a long sunset, the funnel of the headlights revealed just what was necessary to know of the road ahead. My parents talked through the night quietly or not at all, my four-year-old self witness to this dashboard light intimacy.

Eventually I climbed into the rounded window shelf above the back seat and hypnotized myself with the passing lights that faded away into darkness as the radio played softly and my father sang along from time to time. Patsy Cline, Hank Williams, Flatt and Scruggs, music that was always best with a bit of nighttime static behind it conveying great distances, distances already traveled and those left to go.

I was too young to have understood the situations they were singing about in those songs, but the music told me everything I needed to know. The "high lonesome sound" drifted around the car while the hot air poured through my father's window, his elbow languishing on the door. The singer's plaintive storytelling, the Dobro's call, the pedal steel guitar pulling long and low, the fiddle alternating between joy and sorrow—this was life, I came to imagine, or at least my father's idea of life. My mother preferred show tunes with a happily ever after.

I couldn't have explained it until much later, but it was through that car radio I first learned about loneliness and longing and loss, real or imagined. I heard how the music and feeling wrapped around each other in harmony and traveled together with us through the hot night on invisible waves of air.

•

On my first trip alone, I was ten and going by Greyhound to my grandmother's in Miami. My mother reviewed the trip with me several times: sit in the front, get a window seat, hold on to your ticket, and stay on the bus even when it makes the rest stop in Fort Pierce. Grandmom would be waiting at the station downtown, where we would take a city bus to her trailer park.

The driver stowed my little suitcase in the great bus belly, and I climbed aboard with a paperbag bologna sandwich, a book, and a red plastic change purse with a zipper all around and a dollar bill inside. Excitement was the only emotion I felt, although of course excitement is always tinged with fear. My mother told the driver once again where I was going and who would meet me. The Negros were then allowed to board and take their seats in the back of the bus.

The big door whooshed closed, the engine ground into first gear, and the turn signal ticked loudly as we pulled onto the highway. I waved and waved until I couldn't see my mother or the squat cement–block station anymore. The Indian River picked up speed alongside Route 1 as I looked down from high above the passing cars.

At Fort Pierce, the driver announced a twenty-minute rest stop. I got off and walked into the cafeteria. I wasn't afraid. I knew how to order a hamburger and a Coca Cola in a shapely glass with crushed ice and a straw. I knew how to find the restroom and give a nickel to the Negro lady handing out towels. And when the terminal intercom announced: "Port St. Lucie, Palm Beach, Lake Worth, Boca Raton, Fort Lauderdale, Mi-ami," I knew how to find my way back out to the platform and double-check the destination on the front of my bus. I returned to my book and bologna. The bus driver gave me wink as he climbed back into his seat and closed the door.

I left Fishers Island only once that summer of 1969 to go with Mitch and Rob, their sister Carol and her boyfriend George. We piled into George's car at the ferry dock on the mainland and drove to a music festival he knew about in upstate New York. George was the kind of guy who, though not very hip himself, always knew the latest, hippest things—where to get the best weed, or who the up-and-coming bands were that no one else had heard of yet. He already knew this festival was going to be so big you wouldn't even need a ticket to get in.

Woodstock wasn't a place yet in our minds, but the road was, pulling us along with thousands of others to something, someplace, some experience. The Seventeenth Century Japanese poet Bashō said, "The journey itself is home," and it was the journey itself, not the performances of rock's luminaries, that is most memorable for me. The trip became its own home with a traffic jam of epic proportions, surrounded by tens of thousands of people just like us, our new family, our new tribe.

We happily walked the mile or so from where we left the car to carry all our gear (George's gear) alongside our new tribe, which was going to save the world through music, peace, love, and drugs. George had found an old Army tent from his Boy Scout days, and had filled a cooler with over twenty sandwiches—whole wheat peanut butter and jelly, whole wheat hummus and cheese, whole wheat cheese, and three with juicy slabs of ham. A big pot of brown rice still in the pot took up the rest of the room in the cooler.

We felt very self-sufficient in our tent, escaping the confines of the old society. At our neatly laid out site, we even had a couple of folding lawn chairs George had grabbed from his parents' porch. Cool people stopped by to share joints and food. This was what the new world was going to look like, we told ourselves.

By the second night, the tent was leaking, the sandwiches were gone, and the family togetherness was wearing off. Mitch was tripping and morose. Rob was tripping and even more of a loudmouth than usual. George and Carol just made out constantly for two days; rumor had it she was still a virgin. I got tired of wandering around dirty crowds in the mud, having the same boring conversation with different people: "Yeah, it's really cool, man. Yeah, they were fuckin' awesome. Yeah, the outhouses suck."

All those thousands turned out to not necessarily be just like me. But even if they smelled bad and raged on about absurdities and were right in your face, you had to *love* them, as in: "C'mon people now, smile on your brother. Everybody get together, gonna love one another right now."

It was all about sharing, not just sex, but your food and stash and what we would call in the '80s your "personal space." And the only way to turn down *their* offerings, no matter how undesirable, was to say nonchalantly, "I'm cool, man."

In other words, we had to be nice, or we would earn that most terrible of epithets—an uptight chick. I didn't get it. Here we were creating a new society, and we chicks were getting the same message we had gotten when we wore little white gloves in the 1950s—be nice. I didn't want to be nice. I wanted to do my own trip, not somebody else's version of it. I wanted to be on a road that was mine.

•

After the Woodstock summer, I went back to the University of South Florida for a semester, then dropped out. What was the use of going to school when the Revolution was coming? My friend Barbara and I packed up her Plymouth Valiant with all our belongings—our entire record collections in the backseat, including the British version of the first Rolling Stones album. We were going North. Looking at the map laid out on the seat, we decided to go "here"—a spot on the map, the end of the road, the tip of the world, Provincetown. We were beach girls and our homing devices were tuned to the sea and the sand.

Within a couple of days, Barbara and I hooked up with two other young women, Lynn and Dawn, to share a one-bedroom cottage like a treehouse up a long flight of stairs, while we supported ourselves as chambermaids, store clerks, and waitresses. The cottage was actually quite a find, just off the Provincetown main street with all the action but hidden in the treetops.

Our moldy front porch was the perfect place to kick back in one of those uncomfortable old-fashioned metal porch chairs that rusted under the peeling paint, and put our feet up on the railing while the sounds of town drifted up all through the night. We entertained quite a bit there. Ripple wine and weed were usually what we served, and Barbara made a mean macaroni casserole her mother had always cooked with canned tomatoes and ground beef and melted cheese on top.

It was in this cottage on an August night, when there was the tiniest hint in the air that summer wasn't going to last forever, that we came up with our idea. The street was quiet but for Jimi Hendrix singing about being experienced on the record player. Barbara passed me a joint that needed to be re-lit. I could tell it was a Lynn-rolled joint because it was so tight you could hardly get a draw.

"Those dudes with the van were really cool," Barbara said.

"Yeahhh," Dawn said in her usual drawn-out way. "And they *really* appreciated us letting them use our shower."

We all giggled. There had been four of them and four of us in the tiny cottage, although one couple had slipped out to the van.

From below, someone laughed a little too loud, then a glass broke.

"You know," I started. "*We* could get a van like that."

"Why?" Lynn asked. "We scored big with this place, and we've got it the whole summer."

"No, I mean, we could buy a van and travel around like them after the season. They were going all the way to California. We could do that."

"What about our jobs?" Lynn asked. "I'm supposed to be saving my tips for college so my dad doesn't have to give me an allowance."

"A van would be expensive," Barbara added. "Especially one with a rug and stuff like theirs had."

"We could buy it together," I said. "We could all chip in so it would be cheaper. Like the Merry Pranksters or something, a Magic Bus. Only with chicks driving."

"Actually, I think only one person owns the Prankster bus," Lynn mused.

"So?" I was starting to like this idea. "We could all get jobs this winter and save up our money and then chip in on a van for next summer and take off. It would be awesome."

A car went by blasting Bette Midler on its radio. After it passed, you could almost hear the surf off in the distance, a call you knew was there even if you didn't actually hear it.

"Yeahhh," Dawn drawled.

After summer, Dawn and Lynn went back to school, and Barbara and I moved to Boston. In the spring, Dawn called to say she had found a Ford Econoline van with many, many miles on it at a telephone company used equipment sale. We had to act fast to get it, she told me, so I hitchhiked to New Haven to check it out with two hundred dollars worth of savings stuffed into my jeans pocket. Barbara wasn't going; by then, she had decided to move to western Massachusetts to join an ashram.

The boxy van, faded blue like an old police uniform, waited in the back lot of the phone company. On top were rusting matching roof racks for carrying phone equipment. The side door slid open to the empty back, bare except for grooved ridges running up the middle. "They took the radio out," Dawn said, "but that's cool. I hear you can get one installed."

Two seats up front sat on either side of the engine well. Dawn unsnapped the clasps on the engine cover and opened it up. She and Lynn and I stared at the chunk of metal in the well.

"Looks good, doesn't it?" Dawn asked, cracking her gum. We nodded. For six hundred dollars, it was ours, equal shares.

After crisscrossing the country with Dawn and Lynn and a series of boyfriends, I ended up in Northampton, Massachusetts with my then-boyfriend, Charlie. It was three years after Woodstock, and the Revolution still hadn't arrived. The night of Nixon's re-election, Charlie and I were walking home from the bar where we had watched the results on TV. An old Mercury convertible drove by, the top down even on this chilly November night. As it passed, one of the guys yelled, "Four more fucking years!" That pretty much summed up how the world looked to my twenty-two-year-old eyes. The Vietnam War was never going to end; the environment, something we never even knew existed before, was literally going up in flames; the "Silent Majority" made us feel hopeless; and friends were rotting in jails on draft evasion and drug charges.

Other friends, though, were taking action. They were dropping out and going back to the land, even if they had never lived on the land before, to create new societies, more realistic than Woodstock. They were going to use their hands to grow their own food, build their own houses, dig their own water wells, maybe even spin their own yarn from the sheep they raised themselves.

That January after the election, we decided to visit homesteading friends on their farm in Maine. It was already dark by the time we drove over the Piscataqua River Bridge that marked the state line. Our Volkswagen Bug had a heater box you could turn either off or on—the only two choices—until that one day you climbed underneath to change it and realized it was rusted in the wrong position and would be forever. In our case, it was "off," and we had to keep stopping along the way to warm up. Eventually the turnpike dropped us and our rolling tin can into Augusta. We had already been on the road for over five hours and had at least another hour to go.

There wasn't much on Western Avenue in Augusta in 1973. Bolle's Famous for Franks was a bright spot in the darkness, hot and steamy in zero-degree weather. The other customers all seemed to know one another, and there was a friendly solemnity in their interactions. We were clearly strangers there. Our hippy clothes, granny glasses, hair long and uncombed, marked us in stark contrast to the locals who all had gaps between their haircuts and wool plaid collars. But still, it was comfortable, and it seemed a psychic space was made for us when we sat down at the counter. We were all there for the same human reason, after all—food and warmth and maybe a little sign that we weren't alone on a January night.

After warming up and filling up on hot dogs, we drove east on Route 3, mile after mile of darkness with an occasional light from a window spilling over clean, white snow. I tried to read the directions in the faint dashboard light. "Okay, left on Route 220. That was the sign. Should be soon. Slow down."

Charlie aimed the car for the dark strip on the left between the snow banks. The road twisted and turned until it came to a T and we stopped. "This should be the Halldale Road," I said.

We turned left and sure enough within a quarter mile there was an even narrower dirt road going up to the right. To call it one lane between the snow banks would be generous.

"One more mile," I said with satisfaction. But it turned out to be a long and dark mile with some icy patches, the woods seeming to press against our tiny craft. We arrived at what was obviously the end of the road, our friends' driveway circling around the *dooryard* in front of the barn. Dooryard, I thought, realizing I had only read the word before, in those long-ago childhood Florida days spent fantasizing about pioneer life, and now I knew exactly what it meant.

An old-fashioned Maine farmhouse loomed, an attached ell shed running to the barn, everything whitely stark against the night sky. It was after nine and our friends, who had become country folks, had already gone to bed. Charlie turned off the engine we had been hearing grind away for seven hours. It was dead quiet, maybe quieter than I had ever heard before, maybe the same kind of quiet Heidi heard outside Grandfather's hut, the snow and the cold seeming to suck up whatever sound might have ventured forth.

The electric line didn't come up this road, and our friends left a kerosene lantern burning for us inside the ell on the summer-kitchen sideboard. The singular and certain light gleamed on the time-worn wood surface like something out of the Nineteenth Century or a cowboy show. And I knew then I found home, a place where Heidi would feel at ease, a world apart from Space Coast Florida.

CHALLENGER

A clunky metal television set has been rolled into the center of the Belfast High School library. I've brought my class here to break up a day of substitute teaching on a typical gray Maine winter morning. I hadn't realized that today, January 28, 1986, is the day when the space shuttle Challenger, with teacher Christa McAuliffe among the seven astronauts, is scheduled to finally lift off from Cape Canaveral after numerous delays. The television has been pulled out and turned on to follow the launch. My students are poking around the stacks, flirting with each other and pretending to look for books. *Why not watch the launch*, I think, and take a seat.

The usual pre-fight commentary drones on. There is footage of earlier shuttle shots interspersed with a live shot of this huge beast, large and bulky, fuming with liquid oxygen evaporating off its massive body, waiting to be released. Once in a while, the camera pans to a flat stretch of palmetto scrub with a lone cabbage palm stretching skyward and the long open Atlantic as blue as the sky behind it. Another shot shows rows of cars lining the beaches or pulled over to the side of the road with people sitting on the roofs and hoods. Occasionally, the flat voice of the flight director reminds us it is "T minus" however many minutes "and counting."

I hadn't watched a launch in decades. When I left Florida in 1969, my feeling toward rockets was "I couldn't care less," to use a favorite expression of my father's. I didn't pay attention at all to the whole Space Shuttle program that began after I left home. Now, I'm surprised to find myself feeling a tiny bit of the excitement that's been called "that old countdown and liftoff rush."

A few students and the librarian are curious and join me. I turn up the sound as the familiar ten-second countdown begins: Ten, nine, eight, seven, six – "engines are fired" – five, four – "all systems are go" – three, two – "and we have liftoff." There is that moment when it looks as if there is no way this hunk of metal will rise from the smoke and steam. And then the shuttle clears the gantry tower and begins to climb and the camera climbs with it until it is high enough to see traveling through the sky.

The shuttle makes a slight graceful twist as it heads down range, south along the coast, and the flight is turned over to Mission Control in Houston. There is mostly silence as we watch this almost unimaginable spectacle. I am waiting for the first stage to drop off, followed by the small fiery spurt of the booster rockets. More reverent silence, and the television announcer comments in *sotto voce*, "It's a beautiful shot." I am still waiting for the first stage, but I think maybe such things happen differently these days; after all, it's been almost twenty years since I've watched a launch.

Then there is a *large* fiery spurt, which some watching from the beach will think is the boosters, and no one else in the library thinks anything of. But I think, *something is not right. The booster rockets don't make that much of an explosion— at least they didn't use to.* The shuttle disappears inside a white cloud of smoke, *but that could just be the angle of the camera*. Then the smoke plume splits into two different ragged directions, the telltale, sickening sign of a launch gone bad. Houston finally declares that there seems to be "a major malfunction." The flight with so many hopes attached to it has become a disaster. No one in the library says anything. A couple of the girls cry.

A launch gone bad. Along with the horror I just witnessed, I am surprised by another thought: *I can't believe I still know this*. I still know the rhythm of a successful launch. Growing up with the early days of the space program, I know the way it is supposed to look, how much time should pass until that first stage drops off, the arc of success at the beginning of the flight down range, the firecracker fizzle of something gone wrong.

The disaster is a national tragedy, of course, with the deaths of all seven astronauts seventy-three seconds into the flight. Where I come from, it would also be a community tragedy, people we know and most of the Space Coast population connected to it in some way or another. I'm surprised to learn I still feel a tiny part of that community.

SECURITY
CLEARANCE

"Wait here. I have to put my knives in the car to get through security," my brother Ric says.

I have just met up with my brother at the entrance to the Kennedy Space Center. I never like to wait, and I *told him* earlier we'd have to go through security. We are here for "the ultimate journey," as the website says, "where the sky isn't the limit—it's just the beginning." And if that weren't enough, we also have reservations for the special bus tour offered by the Center—"Cape Canaveral Then and Now." But before we can blast off, I have to wait for Ric to drop off his knives.

My little brother, age fifty-six, has a slow, hobbling walk. Maybe it's from decades of carrying seventy pounds of welding equipment a quarter mile to ships in drydock. Or maybe it's from walking the streets of Jacksonville during his junkie days or from a deal gone bad. And he's carrying *knives*—plural?

I can see I'll have a bit of a wait. He and I have parked our respective cars at the far end of the lot. His is the black Lexus, the one he got used "for a very good interest rate," he tells me, at one of those "no credit, bad credit, no problem" places. Mine is the bland rental. It's been over twenty years since the Challenger explosion and I'm here because I've undertaken a research trip to the Florida coast, coming down from my home in Maine to try to re-construct a childhood of wandering the palmettos and watching rockets.

Despite return visits to family most years, I haven't before connected the actual childhood geography with the present one. My re-entry, on the eve of the launch of the final Space Shuttle in 2011, widely considered the end of an era at the Cape, is a conscious return to the landmarks of those early days in which I grew up. With Ric, I've spent the past week visiting my few remaining relatives—my stepfather and the wife he married after my mother died six years ago, my late father's second wife, who I haven't seen in twenty-four years, and Ric from Jacksonville. With Ric, I've visited the East Coast Surf Museum and Ron Jon's Surf Shop, where he could tell me stories about the locally famous surfers in the photos, and later we cruised the docks of Port Canaveral like teenagers sharing a joint with friends.

I want to see where it was my father actually worked during the Fifties and Sixties, an area only open to employees with government Security Clearance. At least, that's why I'm here, and I've invited Ric to come to with me. I could have not mentioned I was going and instead just wandered through the exhibits and my memories alone, quietly taking notes. But I know Ric has a much better memory of the past than I do, so I need his commentary. Ric and I haven't spent this much time together since we were kids and he was known as "Ricky."

As I follow the cement walkway to the Space Center, bland marigolds bloom in evenly spaced rows, and the mild air and warm sun conspire to make it a real Florida tourist "attraction." The swells of welcoming recorded "space" music unfold forever and it feels as if I were actually moving into and through the black and starry great beyond rather than to the ticket booth. I can detect the influences of *2001: A Space Odyssey* in the music. I figure I might as well work on my tan as I wait. I close my eyes and raise my face toward the sun, floating off in the swelling strings of the mood music with no discernible thematic resolution. By the time Ric returns, I am more than ready to get in line at the ticket kiosk and a little edgy from the music.

"Oh shit," Ric says, patting the front pockets of his jeans as we get to the entrance door. "I forgot about the Mace. I have to go back to the car."

"No way!" I say. "Just toss it into that garbage can."

"It costs eight bucks."

"So?"

"I'll stash it in the bushes over there," he points to a cement flower planter attached to the side of the building.

"*What?*"

I look around, hoping no one notices what he is doing. What a hassle it would be to get busted in front of a federal building hiding a can of Mace in the bushes, especially with a two-time felon. I can see how he's made some less than smart choices over the years, and I can't believe he's not extra careful to avoid doing even the tiniest thing that could land him back in jail. As a bit of a careful worry wart, I know I would be.

We're now ready to push our tickets into the machines and walk through the Security Clearance turnstiles. "One at a time," the guard says. I imagine this is something my brother has heard before in other situations involving guards.

We pass through the mysteriously darkened Information Center and wander out into the blazing sunlight of the Rocket Garden. The space music follows. Here, a dozen or so famous missiles, or replicas thereof, stand at attention on cement pads or lie on their sides, each with a little plaque detailing its merits and other factoids about rocket science for those of us who haven't studied rocket science. Mercury, Atlas, Titan, Gemini, Apollo, Saturn, Agena—the names were designed to evoke timelessness and the grandeur of gods.

These missiles are all "old-timers" from the early days of the space industry, the ones launched from the launch pads at the "Old Cape" that we will be visiting. At the Space Center, anything before the beginning of the Space Shuttle program in 1981 is considered ancient history. Some of the rockets have been drawn and quartered to reveal their insides and "stages."

I wander over to one of the smaller rockets and read that it's the Redstone. Ah, the Redstone, a name I haven't heard in thirty-five years. The little plaque tells me that the sturdy Redstone, the workhorse of the 1950s, was drafted into *Project Mercury*, NASA's first manned space program in 1958; this was the year we moved to the area so my father could work at the Cape. *Project Mercury*—how these names come back. Alan Shepard rode the *Mercury 7* as the first American in space, my brother reminds me.

"Oh, right," I say.

"And remember that jump-rope thing you and your friends did?" he asks.

"What 'jump-rope thing'?"

"You know, with the names of the seven astronauts."

I don't remember that because I am trying to remember which one of these corpses my father might have been a part of, or rather I am trying to *imagine* which because I don't think I ever knew. And now there is no one left to ask. I think he was part of the Mercury project, so I look for those with that identification. How could a kid not know what rocket her daddy worked on? Isn't that the kind of thing you'd talk about at the dinner table? Wouldn't you actually get kind of sick of hearing about it every night—assuming he was home every night?

I suddenly remember my father worked in guidance; he was a guidance engineer. Of course, how could I forget? What an ironic job title for him. He wasn't really around the house very much to provide a lot of fatherly guidance, not like those fathers on the TV shows.

I thought I'd come to visit this tourist site to learn more about the space industry for my writing project. Now I realize I'm in search of my father. I am looking for some signs of him I haven't been able to find elsewhere. He has been dead for almost thirty years. I know nothing about his work life, nothing about what he spent his professional career—while it lasted—doing, and what he did all day after he drove the Chevrolet coupe, and later the VW Bug, to join the morning traffic jam on that narrow strip of asphalt out to the Cape.

I asked him once what he did at work. "Draw pictures," he said, joking as usual when he knew I really wanted a serious answer. I figured out later "drawing pictures" had some connection to drafting, in this case, drafting a missile flight plan. He was always the go-to guy at home for math and science projects, and he once explained to me the "rule of thumb" about electrical current, but I don't remember what it is.

As an inheritance, my dad left me a cardboard, twenty-four-can Schlitz beer box, a nice sturdy one with top flaps that tuck in. He presented it to me rather ceremoniously after alluding to it for years. Like most drunks, he was famous for repeating himself, but he was also savvy enough to realize the tragedy and irony that the legacy of a cardboard box represents. He would be the first to admit he was a bit of a failure when it came to fathering and to his career. That didn't mean he would do anything about it.

"That's what you're getting," he would say. As the oldest and the daughter, I would be the keeper of the family heirlooms.

Inside the box were two slide rules in leather cases that he had from his student years, his Navy medals and black leather journal from his days as a flight navigator on an aircraft carrier plane during the war, his diploma in electrical engineering from the University of Miami, and a report card from Thomas Junior High in South Philadelphia. There was a collection of the postcards, two letters, and greeting cards I sent after I left home—maybe fifteen years' worth—although I didn't write much. For a guy who made his career tracking missile courses, his own course was conspicuously untrackable. When I was a kid, his running out for a pack of Chesterfields could mean two or three days with no sign of his whereabouts.

A couple of tourist kids are dashing down the mock gangplank to the mock Apollo capsule, where they can try out the seats. It was this same kind of gangplank that the crew of the *Apollo 1* walked down for the launch dress rehearsal, which ended in an accidental flash fire in 1967, killing the three men. My father wasn't there, I know that. By then, he was out of the industry, never to work at the Cape again. One too many drunk driving arrests and petty misdemeanors meant he lost his all-important, government-issued security clearance. Without it, he could no longer drive past the checkpoint gate to get into the Cape. When did that happen, I try to remember. Sometime in the mid-sixties, sometime when I was in high school. I do some quick math and am shocked to realize that my father was a rocket engineer *for maybe only ten years.*

I appraise the rockets again, this time by launch dates. My brother gives me information, more details than I want to know, about how the missiles work or the peculiarities of some of the components, information he's gleaned from his prodigious reading and watching of the Discovery Channel. He takes a professional interest in the welded joints. The only other visitors in the Rocket Garden besides the kids and their parents are a young couple with shiny new wedding bands who are taking an inordinate amount of photos of each other in front of the rockets.

The Kennedy Space Center is the official name of this tourist attraction, museum, and historical theme park. It sits just outside the *NASA* Kennedy Space Center where the real work of space exploration actually happens. In the early days, all the action was out on the edge of the Cape, until the giant Vehicle Assembly Building and the space shuttle launch pads were built farther inland. The Cape Canaveral bus tour is taking us out to see this "old Cape."

At the bus staging area, no fewer than four guards direct us to the right line. Why are these other people here, I wonder. What can their interest be in these relics? Why would they care that the two things a rocket needs are thrust and guidance? Thrust gets it into the air, and guidance keeps it on its all-important track until it slots into its orbit above the atmosphere.

Standing in line isn't so bad because there is a wall-sized map mural of where we will be going. Maps are about imagination as much as fact for me, and I imagine the empty, green spaces between launch sites are still like the open palmetto scrubland I used to wander as a child.

My father always entered through the South Gate, since Satellite Beach is south of the Cape. Once, for a family outing, he drove us up to the South Gate and stopped. Family members without badges weren't allowed. We gazed for a few moments at the other side, at the acres of palmettos that looked just like the side we were on. Then he ceremoniously turned the car around, and we headed back to Cocoa Beach so we could drive our car along the hard-packed sand, the waves on one side and beachfront joints on the other. We found the right spot to park and unloaded lawn chairs, beach toys, towels, grill, charcoal, marinated chicken parts, chips, beer and sodas. We kids headed for the water with my father, who dove head first into the waves, a feat I wasn't yet brave enough to try. As the evening sky turned pink and orange, Ric and I scouted for driftwood. My father made a shallow pit behind the car to dump the fading hot coals into while my mother put away food. My parents drew their chairs around the fire, and Ric and I sat in the sand. Pieces of the wood were added into the pit to flame and flare in the soft darkness, while my father sang all the verses to "A Fox Went Out on A Chilly Night." The times we managed to do these kinds of outings were among my favorites. I sifted the cool night sand through my fingers over and over again, the back of my hand hot from the fire.

Among the other tourists on the tour bus is a slew of thirty-something Russians. What is their interest in this tour, I wonder. Too young to have experienced the Space Race between their country, or their former country, and us. They are dressed too hip to not recognize a certain postmodern irony in the situation. After all, the thing we most feared when I was growing up was the Russians invading Cape Canaveral. Maybe these young people read about the Space Race in their textbooks and how the U.S. was actually losing until sometime in the late Sixties. That's why there was so much pressure on the Mercury program—to catch up with the Russians and the little dog they sent into orbit.

The bridge arches over the Banana River, and we can look out over the flat expanse of palmetto scrublands surrounding a handful of bare patches with missile sites in the middle of them. We can see the Atlantic stretching to Africa. The guardhouse at the gate waves the bus through since we are all completely security-safe. I wonder if the other tourists are surprised at how much of a wilderness this area really is, less developed than, say, the Disney World complex made of solid cement.

Our tour guide, Dave, tells us that what is now called the Cape Canaveral Air Force Station, or the old Cape, is a mostly natural seventeen thousand acres. Right on cue, we spot a couple of armadillos poking along the side of the road. Dave is sure to let us know about the four species of poisonous snakes and alligators we could see. To me, it's all just beautiful. The sky is as big as I remembered it—like being out on the ocean or in the middle of the Great Plains—and because the weather is on the cool side today, it is bold blue. The gray-green palmettos stretch out consistently the same height as far as can be seen, their rough fronds creating texture against the sky. I suddenly remember the jump-rope rhyme: "Car-penter, Coo-per, Glenn, and Grissom. Schir-ra, Shepard, and Mis-ter Slayton."

Dave is filling us in on many facts that involve numbers—dates, speed, thrust, weight, length, numbers of employees, miles around the earth, dollars. Actually, I don't think he ever talks about money, the trillions of dollars spent over the past fifty years on maintaining our space superiority. I have figured out that the "now" of this "then and now" tour is about drumming up taxpayer interest, support, and patriotism for the projects now in process for the future, maybe playing on nostalgia, like you would about the railroads.

It's widely recognized that this is the end of a particular kind of era for the Space Center, an era that saw space exploration as a major national interest and funding priority. After this final launch of the Shuttle Atlantis, the expectation is that everything will be privatized. The local *Florida Today* newspaper featured an article on the up-and-coming private companies that will launch missiles for their own interests. The article also reminded us that the Space Coast has always seen both boom and bust eras. It's hard for me to differentiate between the industry's fluctuations in fortune and my family's.

Dave is also full of anecdotes about the wild Space Coast life. Ric and I lived through most of them. I find myself wondering, what about the one where my father somehow makes the fifteen miles between Cocoa Beach and our house, skipping the driveway but making a course correction up onto the lawn so that the front bumper of the Chevy just kisses the palm tree before he passes out in the front seat. And how my mother got me up extra early the next morning to go out to the car to try to get him inside before the neighbors woke up. Or how on occasions when he didn't make it to the lawn, my mother bundled us kids off to a neighbor's in the middle of the night so she could drive to bail him out on the mainland. How could Dave miss all that?

Dave mentions Bernard's Surf, the watering hole where the astronauts and press corps mingled. Of course, Dave wouldn't have known that at the bar of Bernard's Surf my father cashed his paycheck—the paycheck that briefly made us, like all the families of Cape engineers, among the highest earners in the state. Dad left the pile of bills in front of him so he could just tell the bartender to "take it out of there and something for yourself." Whatever was left at the end of the night went into his pocket. My mother and he eventually agreed that the check would be mailed from the payroll office right to our house.

Dave paraphrases the "Vegas rule" to say that everyone knew that what happened on the Space Coast, stayed on the Space Coast. I wonder, though, what happens if you actually lived here? Does what happened here just stay here forever?

We are now passing Hanger "S," where the Mercury astronauts prepped for launch, Dave tells us. I don't really care much about astronauts, although it's fun to see a famous building we watched on TV. I think my father met a couple of astronauts, officially at work, but I'm not sure.

What I am most excited to learn, though, is that we are going to—and into—the Launch Complex 26 Blockhouse. I know not everyone can say this, but I have always wanted to go inside a blockhouse, especially one my father might have worked in. They have turned this one into part of the Air Force Space & Missile Museum, the part that can only be accessed by this special, security-cleared tour we are on. Nearby is Launch Complex 5/6 from which Alan Shepard and later Gus Grissom were launched on Redstone rockets.

I'm sure this has something to do with my father. I know he spent time in launch blockhouses. I know, or am pretty sure, he worked on Redstones, at least on the unmanned suborbital missions. Or test firings. Yes, I think he was a test engineer, or maybe that was before he was at the Cape when he worked for Sperry Gyroscopes in Virginia. It's all so confusing, the numbers and names and places and dates and jargon attached to someone's life, especially someone in the space industry, but I think my father was actually here in this blockhouse—or one very like it.

The tour bus stops in front and we are told we can wander at will or follow a docent-led tour. In any case, we'll meet back at the bus in a half hour. And, by the way, this is the last bathroom on the tour. I leap up to get off but am still beaten by a line in the aisle. Ric is calmly waiting for everyone else to go ahead. He has learned some kind of Zen acceptance somewhere along the way that I missed out on.

The Russians are chattering among themselves excitedly as they stoop to peer out the bus windows at the squat, white cement building with the slight igloo hump for a roof, also made of cement. We have already learned that the walls are two-feet thick while the roof varies between five and eight feet. The sun hits me in the face as I make the final step off the bus; I had forgotten how forceful and ubiquitous it is here.

The docent swings open one side of the double blast-doors, a heavily plated gateway to a twentieth century fortress. Like the entrance to a cave, the narrow entryway opens into a small chamber, large enough for a dozen or so people to stand comfortably and now decorated with "cheesecake" style rocket photos, as if they are pretty girls posing for the camera. On either side, doors lead into the two firing rooms, the control rooms where the buttons were *actually pushed* to fire up the engines, I'm excited to note.

We learn that everything in the firing rooms—control panels, equipment, lighting fixtures, wiring paths, paint schemes—are original. The buttons and control handles are cute, looking almost like toys with their rounded, braised-metal edges, shaped and sized for mere twentieth century humans just cutting their first space baby teeth. The black buttons stamped with numbers look like the keys on an old-fashioned typewriter. On the front of the control panels are tiny pullout ashtrays like the one in my father's 1954 Chevy. Inside are cigarette butts—original cigarette butts, the docent tells us. Like a child, I imagine that maybe one is my father's, but then I see it is a Lucky Strike, not a Chesterfield.

Two blue-green slits, like reptile eyes, look out at the launch pads only four hundred feet away. The window glass is comprised of forty-two layers of quarter-inch glass. Forty-two layers of mica-thin glass, carefully laid one on top of the other, then heat-fused into a solid block. Even though I can see through it, the view is fuzzy. Only the big, outlined shape of, say, a rocket, or a man's life might be seen, the hot, fiery blastoff obscuring everything else before the shape slowly rises.

Then I see the Burroughs guidance computer. This one is identical to the two that were installed in the Radio Guidance Center. I associate the words "radio" and "guidance" and "test" with my father; he was a radioman on a Navy plane, after all, and a test engineer at another point. I've heard the word "Burroughs" sometime in the past, the way children hear those grownup words without knowing their meaning and then repeat them knowingly.

I read that these computers were used to control the rockets' flight, using five receiving dishes and transmitting guidance commands back to the rocket. In later years, my father mentioned he had used some of the first computers back in the day, the big clunky kind. Indeed, the docent tells us, "The processing computers on board a Mercury mission are now available in a thirty-dollar wristwatch." I stare at the long, brown metal machine, slowly rusting, but receive no messages from it.

I wander outside, another sleepy Florida afternoon. We have been here more than half an hour, but no one seems concerned. Some of the other tourists are still inside asking questions, while others sit at the benches overlooking this Rocket Garden. The tour guide and bus driver are jawing with a couple of the docents. I walk out into the St. Augustine grass, carefully watching for sticker burrs, and sit down on a chunk of cement. Some kind of bird calls from the palmettos in the late afternoon light.

I try to make up a story, a story not about what was, but a story composed of "what ifs" and "as ifs," a story that makes my father something other than a minor engineer on a big project who drank his way out of a security clearance. In this story he is not the father who didn't come home at night. Instead, he is the kind of father who brought us out here on one of those Saturdays in the 1960s when they briefly opened the Cape so families could see daddy's rockets, a father like one of those on TV who, after coming home from work, dispensed loving guidance to his kids.

Too sappy, I think. It could be just an ordinary story. In it my father would be a regular guy who does his job well, maybe gets singled out from time to time for his good work.

He could still be the hail-good-fellow-well-met kind of guy who others greet in the hall, the fellow who always has a joke or a story. Buck, a great guy, a four-square guy, who maybe in later years the younger men call Mr. Buckmaster, until he tells them to just call him Buck. And at home, he could really play the mandolin, not just a few chords before stopping with a "hee-hee" when he messes up.

"What are you doing?" My brother is suddenly beside me.

"Nothing." I realize this is an answer I have given before when my family interrupts me in the middle of one of my stories. "So what's up with all the knives?" I ask.

"My knives? It's just my pocket knife. And the Leatherman has a little knife on it."

A Leatherman, a pocket multi-purpose tool in case he has to fix something along the way, like our father would have done.

We rejoin the tour group. Dave winds up again. A jackrabbit dashes across the crumbling, nearly abandoned road. We are headed toward the launch pad of the disastrous *Apollo 1*.

"The next stop, folks," Dave says, "is hallowed ground."

FALLOUT

This field trip down memory lane my brother Ric and I are taking is the most time we have spent together in years, decades even. At the wheel, he maintains a non-stop patter, punctuated by indignation, on any topic. We have just crossed the Indian River over the Melbourne Causeway to the beach side of Florida's A1A, our old stomping grounds. Melbourne Beach, Canova Beach, Indialantic, Indian Harbor Beach, and our home town of Satellite Beach. He used to be so quiet; I've always been the talkative one.

Now he talks continually about anything, like the news story about the axe murderer captured on video at the hardware store buying multiple bottles of bleach and big plastic bags similar to the ones they found the bodies in. This is not the kind of thing I'm that interested in, but I say, "Uh-huh." Maybe Ric is just nervous, I think, spending time driving his big sister around, the sister whose approval he used to always want.

We've decided to see our old house, the one where we grew up on Albatross Drive. We moved out in 1968 after our parents divorced and my mother married George, taking us into his larger, more grand ranch house in Indialantic. The selling point for us teenagers was supposed to be that the house sat even closer to the beach than our old one, even though the surf wasn't as good down there. The surfers weren't as cool in that town, either, since they all went to Melbourne High rather than to one of the beach schools, like Satellite or Cocoa Beach. They were more like surfer wannabes, my brother and I sniffed, and he made a deal to ride his motorcycle every morning to Satellite for his last years of school so he didn't have to make any more big changes in his life with a new stepfather.

I lived in my stepfather's house a only few months before I left for college; then a year after that, I left Florida for good, eventually settling in Maine. I accumulated college degrees, a family, a professional life. My brother made it as far as Jacksonville. He rarely showed up when I came down for my annual visit. My mother kept me up to date on his jobs— building swimming pools, running heavy equipment, welding at the Navy Yard. But I could never keep track of his rap sheet, which sentence he was serving for which crime and for which drug. Maybe I just didn't listen too closely when my mother called to tell me the latest.

Ric never did graduate from Satellite High. Instead, he possesses the unconnected fact-strewn detritus of the autodidact, information gleaned from the History and Discovery channels, *Smithsonian* magazine, and his prodigious reading. Most of his talk now centers on the stupidity of other people, like the axe murderer, completely washing over his own shortcomings as a two-strike felon and ex-heroin addict on methadone. I can see it's going to be non-stop on this trip.

Seven-year-old Ricky was sleeping in the other twin bed in my room while his was being painted. We had slept in his room a couple of weeks earlier as mine was becoming a nice lavender. It took longer for paint to dry in those days, especially in the humidity, and the smell of new paint hung thickly, ominously, in the air.

Having my little brother sleep over gave eleven-year-old me the excuse to jump back and forth on the beds before settling down for the night. Much later, I was awakened by the sound of my father's drunken voice down the hall—not an unusual sound. I don't remember what he was harassing my mother about this time, but he was loud enough to wake my brother, too.

"What's going on?" Ricky whispered.

"Daddy came home."

We both lay in our side-by-side twin beds, listening. Even though it was the middle of the night, my father wanted my mother to make him dinner. She had already made us dinner earlier, of course, but Daddy didn't want leftovers. He wanted meatloaf, freshly made meatloaf.

"Where's my dinner, Thelma?" he kept saying in that wheedling, nasty voice he used when he was drunk. "Where's my goddamn dinner?"

"He should have eaten his dinner at dinnertime," my brother whispered knowingly.

I couldn't hear my mother's soft reply but I'm sure she was trying to be reasonable, placating.

"I don't care if the goddamn hamburger is frozen," he threatened. "I want meatloaf—now."

Just go to sleep, Daddy, I thought. *Just go to sleep.*

My mother was saying something.

"Thaw it out!" he slurred loudly.

More quiet talking.

"I don't care how goddamn long it takes. Thaw it out." He threw down the words, his voice meaner than I'd ever heard before, even meaner than that time my mother woke up the next day with a broken wrist.

"Remember when we used to go 'moteling'?" I ask Ric as we drive by the new high rises on the way to Satellite Beach.

"Yeah," he snorts a laugh.

"Moteling" was a game my brother and I invented when I was old enough to drive and he was old enough, probably twelve, to know he was privileged to be cruising with his big sister. It would have been a Friday or Saturday night. My mother must have been home if I got the car. Or maybe she was dating George by then, going out in his red Mustang.

Ricky and I would head to the strip in Cocoa Beach, where there was much more action than in our sleepy town. Moteling consisted of pulling into one of the famous motels along the way, like the Vanguard (named after a rocket) or the Sea Missile or the Holiday Inn, where the astronauts stayed when they were in town. These were all open corridor motels, two stories high with hallways like balconies. We didn't have any two-story buildings in Satellite Beach yet. Each motel had a swimming pool, which always looked more intriguing at night with the underwater lights making it so blue. I would pull into a parking spot pretending we had a room there, and we would get out and run around like the kids we were. Then we jumped back into the car and drove away, as if we had done something to feel guilty about.

"I loved the ice machines," I say, remembering how we would open the big doors and get a fistful of ice to suck or throw at each other.

"Yeah, and those Coke machines where you could get a can for a quarter," Ric says, his voice rising with excitement. Back then the new aluminum cans with pop-tops were more exciting than the old-fashioned bottles.

"And the stairs we ran up and down."

"Remember the guy who came out in his hole-y underwear and yelled at us?"

We both laugh, the smiles lingering. Moteling was a comfort sport for Ric and me, perhaps because most of the time we had spent in motels, the family had still been together and my father was sober enough to drive and to play with us. There had been that extended journey to Dad's temporary job in California when we took in Yellowstone, the Black Hills, Glacier National Park, and made the long drive down the Pacific coast, finally reaching Disneyland. We had also lived in a motel for six months in Cocoa Beach while our cement-block house was being built in the new subdivision. It seemed so cozy, all together in those two rooms with Dad on the wagon in honor of our new life in a new house.

Everything on A1A looks vaguely the same now, but different; there is less open space—in fact, no open space—in between the miles of buildings. Before the first rocket was launched from the Cape in 1958, the area was nothing but palmettos and mosquitoes and miles and miles of empty beach. Since then, a whole world has grown up here around the space industry and tourism, expanding wildly in every direction along this two-mile-wide barrier island.

"Oh look. There's the old Missileman Bar," I say. The place, tucked back from the road in what we now call a mini-mall, used to advertise "strippers" but now features "all-nude pole dancers." I guess they've progressed. Occasionally between the towers of condominiums, a glimpse of the ocean teases and a real sea breeze drifts through.

I tune Ric out as I watch the scenery go by. He's too intense, especially at close range. And even though we share some memories, what else do we share, really? What does it mean to grow up in the same home as someone whose life now is nothing like your own? I noticed last night during dinner at George's how Ric presses his point strongly in a conversation, making himself louder to talk over other people, interrupting heedlessly. Just like our father used to do, I realized, sober or drunk, which made him so obnoxious.

"Why is Daddy yelling?" Ricky asked from his bed. "Why is he being mean to Mommy?"

I didn't say anything. I was too busy. *Just make Daddy go to sleep*, I prayed. *Just make him go to sleep.*

"Linda," my brother insisted. "Why is Daddy yelling?"

"He just is."

I heard the sounds of the freezer door opening and closing and the crinkly, sticky sound of a plastic package of meat being unwrapped. "And just thaw it out, Thelma," he said. "I don't want it cooking until the meat is *thawed*."

I could hear my father making sounds with a glass and a bottle, and my mother going through the motions of cooking. Ricky and I waited quietly, unsure whether it was all over or not.

"You're cooking it, Thelma," Daddy suddenly said in that wheedling voice. "I can smell it cooking. I *told you* not to cook it."

By this time, Ricky and I could smell the sweetish odor of hamburger baking, the first stages when it was still raw but warm, a kind of sickening scent, not good enough yet to make you hungry, not good like my mother's meatloaf usually was.

Ric gets quiet when we pull up in front of Satellite High. I tell a few "happy days" stories, like how marching practice on the hot asphalt lot behind the White Castle hamburger joint as a "Scorpionette" dancer for the school band were the best days of my life. How riding the bus home after a night game with my best friends—the other girls on the dance squad—and the occasional instrumental blasts from geeky band members made me higher than anything I was to later smoke. How—

Ric corrects me a couple of times. "It wasn't a *White Castle*. It was a *Royal Castle*. There were no White Castles in Florida. One time when I was at a *White* Castle up in Georgia..."

We both agree the skinny hamburgers on the gummy rolls were awful as we head back out to A1A. The road is so cluttered with new businesses, neither of us is prepared when the turnoff to our old neighborhood appears suddenly on the left. I wanted to check out the little sandy pullout at the top of the street on the right, my access to the untouristed beach, the place where the world suddenly opened up when I crested the dune, but now there was a Domino's Pizza where the pullout used to be.

As we try to remember who lived where, we exclaim how narrow the street is; we agree it's easy to see how our dad almost drove his car onto the neighbor's front porch that night. We pass the cutoff path to our elementary school, now paved and featuring an anti-drug dealer warning sign.

It's still a rather plain neighborhood of one-story cement block tract houses (four models available), the most modern kind in their era of the squat style of Florida ranch houses.

Ours, the kind that had a jalousie "Florida room," was almost the top of the line, and the attached enclosed garage was a step up from the more proletariat carports of other developments.

The buildings must have been better built than one might assume from the rate at which they were constructed, as they seem to still be in good condition after fifty years. The neighborhood looks more working class than it used to, though; the space engineers' families had moved on. Pickup trucks are now parked on lawns. The rough, wide-leafed St. Augustine grass runs ragged along the street edge. Some of the garages have been turned into living spaces and home-based businesses. There are still almost no trees, just a few scraggly cabbage and palmetto palms with straight barrel trunks and green ruffles on top.

We round the corner and stop two doors down in front of 180 Albatross Drive. It looks much smaller, of course. The little porch—the apron of the cement slab one step up from the grass—looks hardly big enough for me and my dolls, never mind the Moxley girls from down the street with their dolls. The imaginary wagon train we traveled on as hardy pioneer women would never fit into the front yard.

Ric and I comment on how large the three palm trees have grown, even the one the dog chewed down to a nub. In all this time, no one has added any other landscaping, at least to the front yard. The cement-block decorative wall off the end with the attached cement planter looks just like it does in all those photos of us in Easter outfits.

I don't tell any happy days stories here. I can't think of any, although surely there are some. Ric is quiet. I might have imagined people in this kind of situation would say, "Remember the time..." and then laugh knowingly together.

Instead, Ric and I just sit in the car in the middle of the street, two middle-aged people looking to the left.

"All set?" Ric asks.

"Yup," I say. And we drive away.

Some kind of movement started up again in the kitchen, like someone bumping into the dishwasher with a clink against its metal side. "You know what this is, Thelma? This is my belt," Daddy said. "You know what happens when I take off my belt?"

I didn't understand. This was actually a kind of family joke with us kids. "You know what happens when I take off my belt?" he would say in his teasing, fake-mad voice.

"Yeah! Your pants fall down!" we would shout and laugh, and he would look sheepish as if he just heard the joke for the first time. As far as I knew, my father had never hit anyone with a belt before.

But then I heard the sound of leather on a body, not a very hard slap but repeated smacking. At least, that's what I thought it sounded like—like hitting. But that didn't make sense to me. *What's happening?* I don't remember if my mother cried out, but eventually I realized Daddy was hitting Mommy over and over with his belt. I held my breath. *How can he do that?*

I could feel Ricky in his bed, frozen like the hamster always was when the cat came into the room. I suddenly had to go to the bathroom really bad, an inside pressure pushing on my bottom. I worked on stopping the feeling, since I wasn't going to get up. We all knew the same thing: If we were very quiet, it would all go away and be over, all the yelling and bad words and threats. He would fall asleep eventually and it would be over.

Then it was quiet for a while and I let out a long, full breath, the first one since I woke. A breeze rustled the crocus bush outside my window. The insects never faltered in their nightly hymn. But I heard the slapping sound start up again, just not as loud or strong as before. *Oh gee*, I thought, and pulled my breath in.

"Let's go see if the Brugenheisser's fallout shelter is still there," Ric says as we pull away from our old house.

"What fallout shelter? And who were the Brugenheissers?" I ask.

"You don't remember Heidi Brugenheisser? She was a friend of yours. Her father was one of those German engineers who came over after the war and became a citizen so he could work at the Cape. I can't remember her brother's name. It was on Sixth Street, Northeast Sixth. It was one of those above-ground ones."

"Are you sure about this?"

We have reached the end of Albatross Drive and are poking down one of the numbered streets full of stark and plain yards with the grass drying under the brutal sun. Just twenty miles from Cape Canaveral, we would have been a prime target for missiles from Cuba. I have no recollection of a fallout shelter anywhere on the beachside, and as an anxious child always worrying about "what next," I would have loved to have a fallout shelter in our back yard.

"Yeah, yeah," Ric continues. "Remember, the Girl Scouts had a Halloween party in it. And Mom and I came to pick you up, so I got to go inside."

"My Girl Scout troop had a Halloween party in a fallout shelter?"

"Yeah, they decorated it with fake spider webs and everything."

I look over at Ric. How does he remember all these things and I don't? He remembers details about my dance recitals, who said what and when, places we went when we were kids, like to Weeki Wachee Springs, and who was with us. I don't remember half of it. I forgot he was the pitcher on his Little League team—even though they were in the state finals. I forgot he even played Little League for four years. And I certainly don't remember a friend named Heidi Brugenheisser or any fallout shelters. Where was I when I was growing up? I wonder.

This time I heard my mother above the belt slapping. "How do *you* like it? Huh? How do you like it?" her voice warbled through tears, over and over. My eyes darted to Ricky, whose glance grabbed mine at the same moment. I didn't know what to think—*was our mother using the belt on our father?* Even as an eleven-year-old, I could hear that her voice was full of frustration, of impotence, of repressed anger, like the wimpy kid on the playground who finally gets pushed too far and starts flailing wildly. My father was quiet for a change.

"Daddy doesn't even feel it," Ricky said in a soft, proud little-boy voice. But it was still a hesitant little-boy voice, full of questions. He stared at the ceiling.

I was annoyed Ricky could be so dumb. "That's because Daddy's drunk," I said,

"Daddy's drunk?"

"Yeah, he drank too much booze."

My brother didn't say anything else. I didn't either. We seemed to be listening to each other listen. Eventually my father must have passed out somewhere, and the house was silent until I heard my mother moving in the kitchen. She clicked off the oven. The oven door creaked open and she slid the pan across the bumpy metal rack. She pulled open one of the drawers and I heard the rip of wax paper along the jagged box edge. It crinkled as she folded it over the meat. The refrigerator door opened and closed. I heard her turning the lights off one by one, until the last one in her bedroom went out. I heard her lie down. The crickets chirped peacefully outside, and I could breathe now. But it was too late.

Suddenly Ric says, "You know, I couldn't stand the smell of wet paint for years."

"Yeah. I felt the same way about meatloaf cooking," I say, looking out the window for a fallout shelter.

The things I do remember about Ricky, other than the pesky brother parts, the kinds of things my mother would still tell stories about, always involved his inventiveness. Once, before he was even a teenager, he traded his home-made skateboard for a mostly broken-down air conditioner he refurbished for his bedroom, its noisy grind echoing down the hall every night. Then he rigged it and his bedside lamp to a piece of plywood wired with a master switch so he could turn everything off and on from his bunkbed.

But those stories were overshadowed a few years later when my mother came home from work to find him sniffing glue on the Florida room couch, the plastic bag next to him and his voice unnaturally high. Then he and Ricky Haskins broke into the back window of the drugstore in the shopping plaza up the street to steal some kind of drug. Family counseling was ordered, and my brother and mother went a couple of times.

My father refused to go. "I know what they're going to say," he told my mother. "That it's all my fault. It *is* my fault."

I was the golden girl of the family, the smart one, the mouthy but well-behaved one, the star of my dance school who got good grades. Ricky was the picked-on one, constantly harassed by our father, what I would call now the projection of my father's self-loathing.

Over the years after I left home, I would hear dribs and drabs about Ric from my mother, although she and George didn't hear much either—maybe just a middle-of-the-night phone call asking for money for an "electricity bill" that needed to be paid immediately. Years later, those old photos of his little boy buzz-cut always made me sad, too sad to look at. Even though he was always smiling, I would feel a little sick to my stomach, especially after I had my own son. I couldn't recall a picture of him as a happy child.

Ric came down from Jacksonville after our father died. No one really knew how to get hold of Ric in those days so he could be at the hospital at the end, but somehow a message eventually got passed along by his roommate or someone. We gathered at Dad's house—really his wife Mimi's house—although gathered is too formal a word. We were there hanging out in the living room—Grandmom Buck, Mimi, a couple of Mimi's sisters, Ric, and myself with my five-year-old son, Eben. My mother was there, inviting herself to accompany me, but no one had a problem with it; after all, she had known Dad and Grandmom Buck her whole life. She had even cried when I called to tell her he died—almost twenty years after the divorce. "He did it his way," she said, quoting Frank Sinatra. "He always had to do it his way," she sobbed.

Now Ric was playing the prodigal son, arm around my mother and grinning hugely for the camera, answering questions in this chatty way I had never seen before. I couldn't help noticing he disappeared often into the bathroom for periods of time, but everything was good. After all, my mother hadn't seen Ric in several years and she was delighted to find him alive. He had even brought along a big three-ring binder filled with memorabilia of his life as a competitive surfer. It turns out he was the East Coast Champion in the Master's class one year, with sponsorships from major surfboard makers. None of us knew about it.

That night of the meatloaf, I already knew it was too late to change anything, to take back what I had said. I squirmed under the clinging sheets, kicked them off, and lay rigid on my back, not daring to look over at Ricky's bed. Now that we had witnessed this together, it wasn't just my shame anymore. Now it also belonged to a little seven-year-old boy who still sucked his thumb. I felt like I had taken away my brother's innocence by telling him Daddy was drunk.

Big sister that I was, *I told.* I told him what was wrong with our father, *his* father. Daddy acted like that because there was something wrong with him, a reason that might explain some of the sounds Ricky must have heard before, confusing, scary sounds for a kid alone in his bunkbed. But explanation didn't make it better, didn't return us to *before* or move us past it. I told—his daddy wasn't the perfect, strong, smart daddy little boys were supposed to have. It was like I had ripped open his innocence against the sharp edges of that wax paper box.

It was all right for me to know. I was older. I was the girl, the smart girl. I could just wait it out, "what next" hovering like the sickening smell of meatloaf cooking. I felt cold now and pulled the sheet back up.

I could never take it back, I realized, not like those cruel things you might say to your girlfriend and then later say you didn't mean them. I was the big sister Ricky had always believed—and I told. *Smarty-pants Linda. Big mouth Linda.* It was all my fault my little brother now knew about our father. It was all my fault and I could never take it back.

The new Pineda Causeway runs behind the old neighborhood where we look for the fallout shelter on Northeast Sixth. The street itself turns out to have more vegetation on it than the rest of the neighborhood, at least in the backyards. Live oaks and banana trees tower over the one-story houses. Untrimmed crocus bushes scramble along the house sides. The perfect symmetry of a Norway pine shades the corner of one of the driveways.

"We should be able to see the air pipe sticking up over the house," Ric says. "I saw a documentary once on old fallout shelters, and the air pipes on the above-ground ones were over a story high. The program was about these guys who look for old shelters across the country. One of them had been turned into a restaurant. I think it was in Louisiana."

Looking through to the back of a long, brown house with a two-car garage and manicured front planter, we can see something a bit rusty sticking up above it all. "There it is!" we exclaim together like a couple of kids. Ric stops the car and we stare at the house. That just might be an air pipe, we agree— *the* air pipe for a fallout shelter.

STAGE III: RECOVERY

There are three major phases in the recovery operation: location, retrieval, and post-recovery activities.

-HISTORY.NASA.GOV

PALMETTOS

Like an open palm of remembrance with many thin waving fingers, the palmetto's fan-shaped leaves spread three feet across. Its leathery fronds rustle and smack each other in any little breeze, and their quickness to bend and move is one of their defenses. The serrated edges and massing habit make a walk through a stand without a trail a painful experience. Impenetrable for humans except by machete, palmettos' dominance in the natural landscape makes an area wild.

Along this stretch of the Canaveral National Seashore north of the Kennedy Space Center, particularly beautiful specimens mass in front of me, a dusty blue-green consistently the same four-foot height and density. In a land of primary colors, this subtle, soft hue usually gets passed over as dull. Unlike thousands of other native Florida species, no one plants a scrappy palmetto as an ornamental.

But what are palmettos? I wonder. Or what, even, is a single palmetto? Although I clearly remember them, I have never really looked at one as I have today. Palmettos were the "woods" of my childhood imagining, the thing grownups wanted to get rid of, the first thing to go with development. Here and now, though, along the National Seashore and in the Merritt Island National Wildlife Refuge, palmettos are a preserved ecosystem bordering the Space Center.

When I hit the national seashore a few days ago, I was home, ecologically. Here, the brush is thick enough to blanket the land and obscure whatever is on the other side. The possibilities of what is hidden give the road its uplift. On one side runs the steady pound of the ocean and the promise of a beach still wild enough for sea turtles to lay their eggs every spring. On the other side, the Indian River.

It's easy to see how someone first got the idea to weave palm fronds into roofs or hats, I realize, because the plants in front of me have woven themselves into a thick mass that has no beginning and no end, like memory itself. How hard it is to pick out just one palmetto. The thick, hairy trunks actually run prostrate along the ground, growing to seven feet long and sending fronds up, rather than out. Palmettos, I think, would make an excellent place to hide something.

I can see that on the ground level a small animal or a slinking reptile could create pathways, a whole hidden world of imagination and possibility and danger. To the right of me, a spider the size of a saucer has stretched a web from one frond to another. I imagine the two-inch American cockroach, known as a palmetto bug, scurrying along the sand, or a scorpion with its tail raised. Even heavy bobcats and panthers could travel through this world on padded feet, wearing down, over time, a path of least resistance, shouldering their way through the bowing fronds.

Like memory, palmettos are difficult to get rid of. A palmetto stand burns readily, but is actually fire tolerant and will sprout new growth within a week or two of burning, or even hacking. Digging them up is the best way, but the extensive roots run deep, making the project a good deal of work. Bulldozers have been the most popular means over the past sixty years, and I can't guess how many tens of thousands of acres of palmettos have been destroyed over the past century to make way for the Florida of the tourist brochures.

I take the jungle boardwalk trail up to Turtle Mound Shell Heap, the middens left by the Timucuan people over a thousand years ago. From the top, I can see the tepid, still Mosquito Lagoon shimmering in the heat. I look past shorebirds poking in the mangroves and far beyond the nests of bald eagles atop lone cabbage palms.

Off in the humid haze, thrusting out of the wilderness like a blocky beacon visible for miles, sits the fifty-two-story Vehicle Assembly Building, the tallest single-story building in the world, where the stages of the final Space Shuttle were fitted together in 2012. And connecting this landscape from the Everglades to South Carolina, palmettos, as ubiquitous as memory, stitch and hold the thin sandy soil in place.

IF CAUGHT IN A RIP CURRENT, OR: HOW I STARTED WRITING ABOUT GROWING UP IN FLORIDA

Courtesy of the National Oceanic and Atmospheric Administration

1. "Don't fight the current."

   The thing about a rip current is that from the beach, you probably can't see it.

2. "Swim out of the current, then to shore."

   This could take time, decades perhaps.

3. "If you can't escape, float or tread water."

   You don't know where the water will carry you.

4. "If you need help, call or wave for assistance."

   Do you hear me? Do you see me?

ORBITING

My heart continues to pump blood through the sixty-year-old Teflon shunt. I saw it on the sonogram and heard the whooshing and squealing of the valves, like a steam locomotive coming into the station.

The sand and water continue to waltz together under a relentless sun. The sea pounds the beach in winter, whispers in summer.

Somewhere in the vast starry great beyond, Telstar travels on, sending out signals into the vastness, coming from space dust, going to space dust, past the exoplanets, past the farthest edges and more edges beyond that.

From the beach, Mommy and Daddy and Little Brother (all gone now) watch and wave: Hovering like a moon on a warm-blooded night, a small cold body, a farther light, a tiny bit of frozen matter, ambivalent, hesitating still.

beep   *beep*   *beep*   *beep*

ABOUT THE AUTHOR

Linda Buckmaster has lived within a block of the Atlantic most of her life. Born in Miami, she grew up in Space Coast Florida and has been in Midcoast Maine for four decades. Former Poet Laureate of her small town of Belfast, Maine, her poetry, essay, and fiction have appeared in over thirty journals. One of her pieces was a Notable Essay in *Best American Essays 2013* and "Fallout" was nominated for a Pushcart Prize. She has been awarded writing residencies at the Atlantic Center for the Arts, Vermont Studios Center, Kezar Lake in Maine, Landfall Trust in Newfoundland, and Obras Foundation in Portugal. Find Linda online at lindabuckmaster.com.

ACKNOWLEDGEMENTS

Portions of this book first appeared, in slightly different form, in *Saw Palm: Florida Literature & Art; Fantastic Floridas; Burrow Press Review; Solstice Literary Journal; Ars Medica;* and *Upstreet 8.* "Security Clearance" appeared in the anthology *In Season: Stories of Discovery, Loss, Home, and Places in Between* from University of Florida Press, 2018.

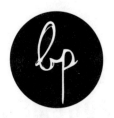

SUBSCRIBE

We thrive on the direct support of enthusiastic readers like you. Your generous support has helped Burrow, since our founding in 2010, provide over 1,000 opportunities for writers to publish and share their work.

Burrow publishes four, carefully selected books each year, offered in an annual subscription package for a mere $60 (which is like $5/month, $0.20/day, or 1 night at the bar). Subscribers are recognized by name in the back of our books, and are inducted into our not-so-secret society: the illiterati.

Glance to your right to view our 2018 line-up. Since you've already (presumably) read *this* book, enter code **SPACE25** at checkout to knock 25% off this year's subscriber rate:

BURROWPRESS.COM/SUBSCRIBE

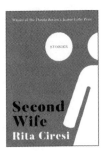

Second Wife
stories by Rita Ciresi
978-1-941681-89-3

Linked fictional snapshots of feminine lust, loss and estrangement by the Flannery O'Connor Award-winning author of *Mother Rocket*.

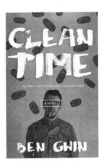

Clean Time: the True Story of Ronald Reagan Middleton
a novel by Ben Gwin
978-1-941681-70-1

A darkly comic satire of academia, celebrity worship, and recovery memoirs set in a near-future America ravaged by addiction.

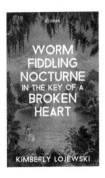

Worm Fiddling Nocturne in the Key of a Broken Heart
stories by Kimberly Lojewski
978-1-941681-71-8

Fabulist, folkloric and whimsical stories featuring an itinerant marionette, a camp counselor haunted by her dead best friend, and a juvenile delinquent languishing in a bootcamp run by authoritarian grandmas… to name a few.

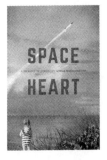

Space Heart
a memoir by Linda Buckmaster
978-1-941681-73-2

The story of growing up in 1960s Space-Coast Florida with a heart condition and a, rocket engineer father.

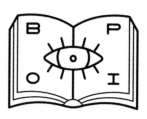

the illiterati

Florida isn't known as a bastion of literature. Being one of the few literary publishers in the state, we embrace this misperception with good humor. That's why we refer to our subscribers as "the illiterati," and recognize them each year in our print books and online.

To follow a specific publishing house, just as you might follow a record label, requires a certain level of trust. Trust that you're going to like what we publish, even if our tastes are eclectic and unpredictable. Which they are. And even if our tastes challenge your own. Which they might.

Subscribers support our dual mission of publishing a lasting body of literature and fostering literary community in Florida. If you're an adventurous reader, consider joining our cult—er, cause, and becoming one of us...

One of us! One of us! One of us!

2018 illiterati

Emily Dziuban
John Henry Fleming
Nathan Andrew Deuel
Dina Mack
Abigail Craig
Teresa Carmody
Spencer Rhodes
Stephen Cagnina
Letter & Spears

Matthew Lang
David Rego
Rita Sotolongo
Michael Wheaton
Thomas M. Bunting Projects
Michael Cuglietta
Christie Hill
Alison Townsend
Rick Gwin & Peggy Uzmack

Michael Gualandri
Hunter Choate
Nathan and Heather Holic
Rita Ciresi
Drew Hoffmann
Lauren Salzman
Joanna Hoffmann
Dustin Bowersett
Stacey Matrazzo
pete !
H Blaine Strickland
Karen Price
Leslie Salas
Jessica Penza
Randi Brooks
To a Certain Degree
Yana Keyzerman
Erica McCay
Alexandra Mariano
A.G. Asendorf
Sarah Taitt
Winston Taitt
Lauren Zimmerman
Martha Brenckle
Nikki Fragala Barnes
Michael Barnes
Matthew Broffman
Shaina Anderson
Stuart Buchanan
Shane Hinton
Cindy & Frank Murray
Suzannah Gilman
Anonymous
The Huntress Bird Sanctuary

Allie Marini
Matt Lonam
Naomi Butterfield
Peter Bacopoulos
Ted Greenberg
Gene Albamonte
Erin Hartigan
Sean Ironman
Victoria Elizabeth Webster-Perez
Danielle Kessinger
Susan Lilley
Kim Britt
Janna Benge
Kara Black
Rebecca Evanhoe
Vicki Entreken
Jeff Parker
The Noel Family
Cooper Levey-Baker
Aileen Mulchrone
David James Poissant
J.C. Carnahan
Heather Owens
Stacy L. Barton
Whatever Tees
Nayma Russi
Lauren Mitchell
Roberta Alfonso
Terry Godbey
Bob Morris
libby ludwig
Mary T. Duerksen
Kana Philip
Debbie Goetz

MORE FROM BURROW PRESS

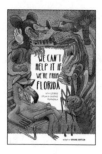

We Can't Help It If We're From Florida
ed. Shane Hinton
978-1-941681-87-9

"As hot and wild and dangerous as our beloved (or is it bedeviled?) state, itself."
–Lauren Groff, *Fates & Furies*

"As weird and funny and beautiful and unnerving as you might expect from some of our state's best writers." –Karen Russell, *Swamplandia!*

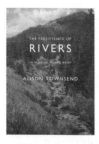

The Persistence of Rivers: an essay on moving water, by Alison Townsend
978-1-941681-83-1

In the vein of Thoreau and Dillard, Townsend considers the impact of rivers at pivotal moments in her life, examining issues of landscape, loss, memory, healing, and the search for home.

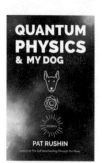

Quantum Physics & My Dog Bob
stories by Pat Rushin
978-1-941681-81-7

Each darkly funny story is like a parallel universe where everyday characters find themselves in a reality slightly askew from the one we know.

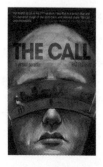

The Call: a virtual parable
by Pat Rushin
978-1-941681-90-9

"Pat Rushin is out of his fucking mind. I like that in a writer; that and his daredevil usage of the semi-colon and asterisk make *The Call* unputdownable."
–Terry Gilliam, director of *The Zero Theorem*

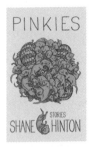

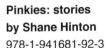

Pinkies: stories
by Shane Hinton
978-1-941681-92-3

"If Kafka got it on with Flannery O' Connor,
Pinkies would be their love child."
– Lidia Yuknavitch, *The Small Backs of Children*

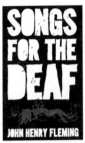

Songs for the Deaf: stories
by John Henry Fleming
978-0-9849538-5-1

"Songs for the Deaf is a joyful, deranged, endlessly
surprising book. Fleming's prose is glorious music;
his rhythms will get into your bloodstream, and his
images will sink into your dreams."
– Karen Russell, *Swamplandia!*

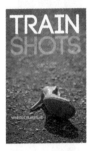

Train Shots: stories
by Vanessa Blakeslee
978-0-9849538-4-4

"*Train Shots* is more than a promising first
collection by a formidably talented writer; it is a
haunting story collection of the first order."
– John Dufresne, *No Regrets, Coyote*

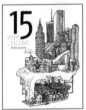

15 Views of Miami
edited by Jaquira Díaz
978-0-9849538-3-7

A loosely linked literary portrait of the Magic
City. Named one of the 7 best books about
Miami by the *Miami New Times.*

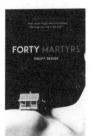

Forty Martyrs
by Philip F. Deaver
978-1-941681-94-7

"I could hardly stop reading, from first to last."
– Ann Beattie, *The State We're In*

MORE FROM FLORIDA

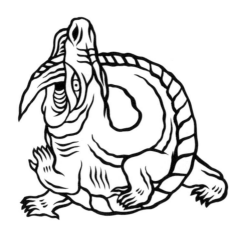

FANTASTIC FLORIDAS

Taken out of context from a mediocre translation of Rimbaud's poem, "The Drunken Boat," Fantastic Floridas is Burrow Press' weekly online journal featuring new fiction, essays, poetry, interviews, excerpts, art & et cetera.

BURROWPRESS.COM/FLORIDA